100 Questions & Answers About Lymphedema

Saskia R. J. Thiadens, RN
National Lymphedema Network, Inc.
Oakland, CA

Paula J. Stewart, MD, CLT-LANA
Division of Lymphedema Services
Medical Director
Lakeshore HealthSouth
Birmingham, AL

Nicole L. Stout, MPT, CLT-LANA
Physical Therapist and Lymphedema Specialist
National Naval Medical Center Breast Care Center
Bethesda, MD

JONES AND BARTLETT PUBLISHERS
Sudbury, Massachusetts
BOSTON   TORONTO   LONDON   SINGAPORE

World Headquarters
Jones and Bartlett
  Publishers
40 Tall Pine Drive
Sudbury, MA 01776
978-443-5000
info@jbpub.com
www.jbpub.com

Jones and Bartlett
  Publishers Canada
6339 Ormindale Way
Mississauga, Ontario L5V 1J2
Canada

Jones and Bartlett
  Publishers International
Barb House, Barb Mews
London W6 7PA
United Kingdom

Jones and Bartlett's books and products are available through most bookstores and online book-sellers. To contact Jones and Bartlett Publishers directly, call 800-832-0034, fax 978-443-8000, or visit our website, www.jbpub.com.

Substantial discounts on bulk quantities of Jones and Bartlett's publications are available to corporations, professional associations, and other qualified organizations. For details and specific discount information, contact the special sales department at Jones and Bartlett via the above contact information or send an email to specialsales@jbpub.com

The authors, editor, and publisher have made every effort to provide accurate information. However, they are not responsible for errors, omissions, or for any outcomes related to the use of the contents of this book and take no responsibility for the use of the products and procedures described. Treatments and side effects described in this book may not be applicable to all people; likewise, some people may require a dose or experience a side effect that is not described herein. Drugs and medical devices are discussed that may have limited availability controlled by the Food and Drug Administration (FDA) for use only in a research study or clinical trial. Research, clinical practice, and government regulations often change the accepted standard in this field. When consideration is being given to use of any drug in the clinical setting, the health care provider or reader is responsible for determining FDA status of the drug, reading the package insert, and reviewing prescribing information for the most up-to-date recommendations on dose, precautions, and contraindications, and determining the appropriate usage for the product. This is especially important in the case of drugs that are new or seldom used.

The views expressed in this book are those of the author(s) and do not necessarily reflect the official policy or position of the Department of the Navy, Department of Defense, nor the U.S. Government.

Production Credits
Executive Publisher: Christopher Davis
Editorial Assistant: Sara Cameron
Associate Production Editor: Leah Corrigan
Senior Marketing Manager: Barb Bartoszek
V.P., Manufacturing and Inventory Control: Therese Connell
Composition: International Typesetting and Composition
Cover Design: Carolyn Downer
Cover Images: © Photodisc, © John Sartin/ShutterStock, Inc., © Tan Wei Ming/ShutterStock, Inc.
Printing and Binding: Malloy, Inc.
Cover Printing: Malloy, Inc.

Library of Congress Cataloging-in-Publication Data
Thiadens, Saskia R. J.
   100 questions and answers about lymphedema / Saskia R.J. Thiadens, Paula J. Stewart, Nicole L. Stout.
       p. cm.
   ISBN 978-0-7637-4989-7 (alk. paper)
   1. Lymphedema—Miscellanea. I. Stewart, Paula J. II. Stout, Nicole L. III. Title.
   IV. Title: One hundred questions and answers about lymphedema.
   RC646.3.T45 2010
   616.4'2—dc22
                                                                        2009025799
6048

Printed in the United States of America

13 12 11 10 09   10 9 8 7 6 5 4 3 2 1

This book is dedicated to all people with lymphedema and to their loved ones who are affected by lymphedema. It is for every committed therapist and physician who provides care to people with lymphedema, as these providers go above and beyond to help their patients manage and understand their condition. Our common goal and sincere hope is universal recognition and treatment for this disease.

Contents

This book by Saskia Thiadens, Nicole Stout, and Dr. Paula Stewart offers a transparent, practical orientation for doctors and therapists, but is primarily aimed at patients. Structured as 100 questions and 100 answers, the imparting of information has been masterfully achieved—a kind of patient-guideline—in order to prevent and treat lymphedema, and thus improve quality of life. We can only thank the authors and congratulate them on this book! We hope that it will reach as many lymphedema patients and those at risk of developing the disease as possible.

Etelka Földi, *MD*
Földiklinik
Hinterzarten, Germany

Acknowledgments

We would like to thank those whose help was integral to the production of this book. Joachim Zuther, who assisted us with obtaining diagrams and glossary terminology. Bonnie Pike and Jan Hasak for their contributions as patients; we must never forget what they face in dealing with this condition on a day to day basis, their input and perspectives here within are invaluable to the medical provider. Dr. Etelka Földi for graciously agreeing to write the foreword. To our professional colleagues, from whom we learn something new every time we interact. To our family, friends, and loved ones.

PART ONE

The Basics

Are there different types of lymphedema?

What are the common causes of lymphedema?

How do I get lymphedema treated or cured?

More . . .

1. What is lymphedema?

Lymphedema is an abnormal swelling condition that may affect one or many body regions. The swelling develops because the lymphatic vessels or nodes have been damaged or were formed incorrectly. Lymphedema is most commonly a side effect of cancer treatments. If a person has surgery to remove **lymph nodes**, as is common for cancer treatment, or if they have radiation for cancer, the damage done to the **lymphatic system** may result in a back-up of fluid. The lymphatic system is the body's plumbing system and is responsible for removing waste material from the body. Just as you would imagine, if the plumbing system in your home were disrupted or damaged, you may end up with a back-up of waste. The same is true in your body. The back-up of waste products from the cells in the body, along with water and protein, builds up in your tissue and causes swelling to occur (**Figure 1**).

Lymph node

One of the many small oval structures that filter lymph and fight infection.

Lymphatic system

A vast, complex network of capillaries, thin vessels, valves, ducts, nodes, and organisms that help protect and maintain the internal fluid environment of the entire body by producing, filtering, and conveying lymph and by producing various blood cells.

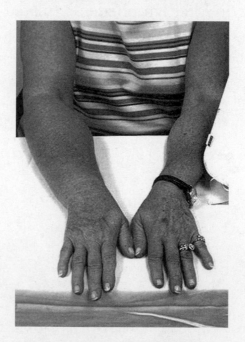

Figure 1   Unilateral upper extremity lymphedema.

Lymphedema can be from many different causes. Some lymphedema occurs because the lymphatic system was damaged with surgery or another trauma. This is called secondary lymphedema and is the most common type of lymphedema. Sometimes people are born with a condition that causes the lymphatic system to not work correctly. This is called primary lymphedema. Both types of lymphedema can affect any part of the body where lymphatic vessels have been damaged or malformed.

When the swelling occurs in the body, and is not treated it can get worse over time. As the swelling worsens, changes occur in the tissue, resulting in scarring and hardening of the tissue. Also, as the waste products back up into the tissue, there is an increased risk of infection because the body cannot process and eliminate the bacteria that it is encountering in the area where the damage has occurred to the system.

While lymphedema can be treated to decrease the swelling, and while relapses of swelling can be prevented, there is no cure for lymphedema. The condition involves lifelong management of the swollen limb(s) with complete decongestive therapy (CDT) to decrease the swelling and to prevent adverse side effects like infections and skin breakdown.

2. What are lymphatics and lymphatic vessels?

Lymphatics are an intricate network of vessels and nodes found throughout the body. Lymphatic vessels are responsible for absorbing the protein-rich fluid and waste products from body tissues and transporting that fluid away from the tissue. The lymphatic system also contains lymph nodes, which filter and clean the fluid. Filtration through the lymph nodes is important for removing

Lymph

A thin, watery fluid originating in organs and tissues of the body that circulates through the lymphatic vessels and is filtered by the lymph nodes. Lymph enters the bloodstream at the junction of the internal jugular and subclavian veins.

waste products, such as bacteria, from the **lymph**. Bacteria and other waste products are strained out by the node and held there until the body's immune system can naturally break down and eliminate this waste.

The system begins with vessels found just below the surface of the skin. These vessels are called lymphatic capillaries and are responsible for absorbing fluid from the tissue and bringing it into the vessel network. Lymphatic capillaries are thin and delicate. The fluid then passes through a network of larger vessels called lymphatic collectors, which bring the fluid into the more central regions of the body. The lymph collectors are larger, thicker vessels responsible for transporting the fluid. The collectors contain a sequence of valves, distributed at intervals within the vessel, which guide fluid flow in a specific direction. This directed flow is important to prevent backflow of lymphatic fluid.

Lymphatic collectors have a layer of muscle within the vessel. When the muscle of the vessel is stimulated by the fluid filling it up, a contraction occurs and the vessel pushes the lymphatic fluid through the system. This important process is the primary way the system works to move fluid. The lymphatic system does not have a central pump, like the heart, to force fluid through the vessels; therefore, this internal muscle contraction is the most important process to move fluid through the system.

Lymphatic fluid comes from the body tissues and is comprised of water, fat cells, proteins, and white blood cells. Also, any waste products produced by our cells along with bacteria or viruses that our body encounters will be carried in the lymphatic fluid. These waste materials have to be filtered out of the lymph fluid before the fluid can be returned into the rest of the body.

Our bodies contain over 500 lymph nodes. They are distributed throughout the body and are commonly found in clusters. Large clusters of nodes are found in the abdominal area, the neck, the armpits, and the groin. When lymph nodes have a large amount of waste products to handle, such as when you experience a cold or a fever, they may become enlarged and sometimes are tender. The lymphatics are working harder than usual because they are overburdened with handling the bacteria that caused your illness. As your body heals itself from the illness, it will naturally break down and eliminate these bacteria. However, there are times when the lymph nodes become full of cells that the body cannot naturally break down, such as cancer cells. If you feel lymph nodes that are enlarged and they do not get smaller after your illness subsides, or if the nodes are enlarged when you have not been ill, you should consult with your doctor to determine if the nodes need to be investigated further.

Bonnie says:

What a surprise the lymphatic system is! Everybody's heard of the circulatory system, the nervous system, the digestive system, or the skeletal system, but who ever gives any thought to their lymphatic system? Not me. At least not until my lymphedema diagnosis. Then I had to hurry up and learn all the new words and concepts that go along with this practically invisible body system. At first it was simply confusing, and I felt intimidated by all the terms I didn't understand. But learning what the lymphatic system is and how it works is important to being able to manage

If you feel lymph nodes that are enlarged and they do not get smaller after your illness subsides, or if the nodes are enlarged when you have not been ill, you should consult with your doctor.

it when it's broken—like mine is. So I read everything I could about it and asked lots of questions. Now I think of it with awe for all the things it does to protect us from infection and disease.

3. Are there different types of lymphedema?

Yes, lymphedema may arise from a variety of reasons and may occur in any body region. While there are many different types of lymphedema, the one thing that all types have in common is that they involve a back-up of protein-rich fluid in a region of the body. The two main types of lymphedema are primary and secondary.

Congenital

A condition that is present at birth or very shortly after birth.

Hereditary

Pertaining to a genetic characteristic transmitted from parent to offspring.

Hypoplasia

A decrease in the number of lymphatic vessels or nodes that are formed so that they are unable to handle processing a regular volume of lymphatic fluid.

Hyperplasia

Growth of lymphatic vessels that are too large to be functional. The vessels are so large that their ability to move fluid is impaired.

Aplasia

The absence of lymphatics. Used to reference a region of the body where lymphatic nodes or vessels failed to develop or grow.

Primary lymphedema is the result of a **congenital** or **hereditary** condition that affects how the lymphatic vessels are formed. In some people, the condition is congenital, or present at birth or very shortly after. In some, the condition does not present until later in life such as during puberty, or even later. Primary lymphedema may result from a **hypoplasia** of lymphatic vessels (a decrease in the number of lymphatics formed), a **hyperplasia** of lymphatic vessels (vessels that are too large to be functional), or an **aplasia** (absence) of lymphatics. Many different types of primary lymphedema exist. Some of the most common types are Nonne-Milroy's disease, Meige's disease, and Distichiasis syndrome.

Secondary lymphedema occurs when there is an incident that causes trauma to the healthy lymphatic system and damages it. In secondary lymphedema, there is typically a known cause for the lymphatic system's damage. Common causes of secondary lymphedema are surgery involving lymph node dissection, radiation therapy, traumatic injury, **post-thrombotic syndrome**, and filarial infection (see Question 4).

4. What are the common causes of lymphedema?

In the United States, 90% of all lymphedema is caused by trauma to the lymphatics. Most of this occurs with surgery, especially cancer surgery where removal of lymph nodes is routinely performed to determine if the cancer has started to spread to other regions of the body. With the removal of lymph nodes, there is often scarring of the remaining lymphatic vessels, which results in a barrier preventing fluid removal from the distant areas of the body and subsequent swelling in the affected tissue. For example, more than 20% of those undergoing a modified radical mastectomy (MRM) and lymph node removal will develop lymphedema.

Radiation therapy, related to cancer treatment, can also result in lymphedema. Radiation causes scarring and **fibrosis** of the lymphatics located within the radiation field, making it more difficult for the vessels to function adequately, sometimes resulting in lymphedema. It is reported that an MRM along with radiation therapy is associated with a greater than 30% risk of developing lymphedema. Radiation will also prevent regrowth of new lymphatics (**lymphangiogenesis**). The effects of radiation therapy may occur long after the treatment has ended. Even years later, there may be continued scarring and fibrosis to the tissue related to past radiation treatment. As injury to the lymphatics accumulates over this time without a means of repair, the affected limb may become more susceptible to the onset of lymphedema. This disease process may be why we sometimes see lymphedema start many years after cancer treatments are completed. For more on radiation therapy, see **Box 1**.

The Basics

Post-thrombotic syndrome

A complication that may follow a deep vein thrombosis (DVT) and includes symptoms such as persistent swelling, pain, bruising of the skin, eczema-like skin changes, itchiness, and infections. Also called post-phlebitic syndrome.

Fibrosis

Scarring of the soft tissue of the body. In lymphedema, the scarring is caused by long-standing lymph fluid congested in the tissue.

Lymphangiogenesis

The formation of lymphatic vessels from preexisting lymphatic vessels. When a tumor grows in the body, it signals the lymphatic vessels to grow new vessels.

| BOX 1 | *The Field of Radiation Therapy: Why Are We Concerned with It?* |

Radiation therapy is the delivery of ionized particles to a body region in an effort to kill any remaining cancer cells. The treatment, however, has an impact on all of the surrounding tissue in the field where radiation is delivered. Treatment results in significant inflammation of the tissue. During treatment the tissue may become very red, warm to the touch, and tender. Once treatment has finished, these acute symptoms will go away; however, there are some symptoms that will remain.

The radiation field includes all of the tissue that the radiation beams target for treatment. How do you know where the field is? Sometimes after radiation therapy, the skin remains slightly altered in its color as compared to the surrounding skin. Every patient receiving radiation has been given small tattoos that look like tiny dots on the skin. These dots outline the field that is treated. You can identify the field by finding the dots. Identifying the field is very important and helps to guide your medical team in recommending the safest treatment for you.

Cellulitis

An acute infection of the skin and soft tissue, usually caused by bacteria, characterized by local heat, redness, pain, and swelling, and occasionally by fever, malaise, chills, and headache.

Lymphangitis

An inflammation of one or more of the lymphatic vessels, usually resulting from an acute streptococcal infection of one of the extremities.

Edema

Swelling that is caused by the accumulation of watery fluid in the soft tissues, joint spaces or body cavities.

Another frequent cause of secondary lymphedema in the United States is severe tissue trauma, such as that sustained from motor vehicles crashes, work-related injuries, falls, sports injuries, and household accidents. Any time the lymphatics are damaged or scarred, there is a risk of developing lymphedema. Lymphedema can also occur after infection, as with **cellulitis**, an infection involving the tissue, or **lymphangitis**, an infection involving the vessels.

Other types of **edema** can occur from multiple causes and contribute to the development of lymphedema.

Post-thrombotic edema refers to the swelling associated with a deep venous thrombosis (DVT), which is a blood clot in a vein. The blood clot will cause scarring in the wall of the vein and results in slowing or blockage of venous blood flow. This may result in a back-up and pooling of blood. When this pooling is mild, varicose veins on the limb result; however, if the blood pooling becomes chronic, swelling may occur in the limb.

The most common cause of lymphedema in the world is filarial disease. This mosquito-born parasite plagues tropical regions of the world and infects over 300 million persons. For more on filariasis, see **Box 2**.

The most common cause of lymphedema in the world is filarial disease.

BOX 2	*Filariasis and Filarial Infections*

In the subtropical areas of the world, a filarial infection is the leading cause of lymphedema. What is **filariasis**? It is a condition where a worm grows inside of the lymphatic system and causes destruction of the healthy vessels and nodes. The worm gets there when a mosquito carrying the eggs (larvae) of the worm bites a human and transmits the eggs. These mosquitoes only live in areas such as the tropics—Central and South America, South Asia, Tropical Africa, and some of the Caribbean islands.

When the mosquito bites a human, it transmits the larva into the bloodstream. The larva travels to the lymphatic system where it grows into an adult worm. The adult filarial worm then lays eggs in the lymphatic vessels and therefore promotes ongoing growth and spread of the worms throughout the system. Growth of the worms takes from 3 to 12 months.

(*continued*)

Filaria

A long, thread-shaped worm. In humans, they may infect the lymphatic vessels and lymphatic organs, circulatory system, connective tissues, subcutaneous tissues, and serous cavities.

Filariasis

A chronic disease caused by the parasitic nematode worm *Wuchereria bancrofti* or *Brugi malayi*. The worm lives and grows in the lymphatic vessels, making them unable to move fluid and resulting in lymphedema.

BOX 2 *(Continued)*

The worms block the flow of lymph fluid through the vessels and also damage the vessels, leaving them unable to carry lymphatic fluid. This results in a backup of protein-rich fluid in the tissues of the body and the swelling that causes lymphedema. As you can imagine, the condition will continue to progress until the worm dies and is unable to reproduce. Filariasis is the leading cause of lymphedema worldwide.

Treating filariasis has become a prominent goal of the World Health Organization (WHO). The WHO Global Program to Eliminate Lymphatic Filariasis has two goals. The first goal is to stop the spread of infection by filarial worms. This is accomplished by delivering special medications to the population "at risk." The WHO has teamed with numerous organizations worldwide to obtain and distribute Ivermectin to populations at risk. This drug prevents the spread of the condition. It is given in a single dose, yearly, for 4–6 years. The second goal of the WHO program is to alleviate the suffering of affected individuals. Treating lymphedema in these settings is often challenging. The treatment for filarial lymphedema is exactly the same as the treatments we use here in the United States. However, since most of the countries impacted by filariasis are poor, third-world countries, the resources and supplies needed to adequately treat and maintain lymphedema are not readily available. Ongoing efforts by organizations such as GlaxoSmithKline, Merck Inc., The Gates Foundation, and the Global Alliance to Eliminate Lymphatic Filariasis are contributing to achieving these goals.

In the United States, 10% of all lymphedema cases are primary and due to congenital or inherited deficiencies of the lymphatics. The most common primary deficiency in the lymphatic system is not associated with a specific hereditary condition (such as Milroy's or Meige's diseases) but is related to a general lack of lymphatic collectors. This anomaly will typically result in swelling of the lower extremities. When it occurs before an individual is 35 years old, it is called lymphedema praecox. Vessel anomalies in the lymphatic system may also present later in life. If the condition arises after the age of 35 years, it is then called lymphedema tarda. These terms—lymphedema praecox and lymphedema tarda—are the diagnoses given to the majority of cases of primary lymphedema in the United States.

Some cases of primary lymphedema are due to an absence of lymphatics associated with a specific genetic condition (see Question 86). When this condition occurs, and an infant is born with lymphedema, it is called Milroy's disease. Other conditions that may present later in life, such as Meige's disease, are also responsible for lymphedema. Other genetic conditions associated with lymphatic abnormalities include Noonan's syndrome, Turner's syndrome, Klinefelter's syndrome, and many others. There are dozens of genetic anomalies that include lymphedema as a part of the syndrome, and an exhaustive list cannot be accurately provided here. The commonality among these conditions is that they cause lymphedema from a genetic abnormality that diminishes the number of functional lymph vessels in the body.

In rare instances, primary lymphedema is due to hyperplasia of lymphatics, which is when the vessels are super-sized. The vessels then are too large to function correctly. When this occurs, the valves within the collector vessels are unable to help the body propel fluid away from the tissue, resulting in a back-up of fluid and eventually in swelling. This condition is often associated with other genetic anomalies.

5. Why do they have to remove lymph nodes? And am I at a greater risk if more are removed?

The removal of lymph nodes is an essential part of diagnosing and treating cancer. Lymph nodes are removed from the area of the body where the tumor is located and help to determine if the cancer cells have started to spread throughout the body. Not all cancers are assessed by removing lymph nodes, but the majority are; therefore, removal of lymph nodes is an important part of treating cancer. Since the lymphatics do not have the ability to regrow after they are removed or damaged, the capacity of the system to move fluid and waste products is decreased whenever vessels or nodes are removed. Again, just like your plumbing, if more plumbing is removed, the risk for a back-up is greater.

Melanoma

Any of a group of malignant neoplasms, primarily of the skin, that are composed of melanocytes.

The sentinel lymph node biopsy, which is a lymph node-sparing technique used with breast cancer and some types of **melanoma**, can greatly reduce the risk of developing lymphedema. The sentinel node biopsy involves taking only a small number of nodes rather than a full dissection, which may take as many as 40 nodes. Having more lymph nodes removed does mean that your risk for developing swelling in that area of the body is greater. For more on sentinel lymph node biopsy, see **Box 3**.

| BOX 3 | *Sentinel Lymph Node Biopsy: Changing the Risk Factors* |

The sentinel lymph node biopsy (SLNB) is a procedure used to selectively remove lymph nodes during cancer surgeries. The technique is used during either a lumpectomy or mastectomy surgery. The sentinel node is identified by injecting both a blue dye and a small amount of radioactive material into the tissue near the tumor and mapping which lymph node it travels to first. That first lymph node(s) (there may be up to three) is removed and checked during the surgery for evidence of cancer invasion. If no cancer cells are found, no other lymph nodes are removed. If cancer cells are found, then a full lymph node dissection is performed and typically 15 to 30 lymph nodes are removed.

The SLNB has helped to reduce many of the complications associated with cancer surgeries. Remember that lymph node removal is a risk for developing lymphedema, so taking less lymph nodes out greatly reduces the risk. SLNB is being routinely used in breast cancer, head and neck cancers, and melanoma.

The Basics

6. What if I have never had lymph node surgery? Can I still get lymphedema?

As discussed in Question 4, lymphedema can occur without surgery in several instances. The most common cause of lymphedema worldwide is filarial disease, where lymph nodes become infested with worms that grow from a parasite that is transmitted by mosquitoes (see Box 2). In the United States, surgery is the most common cause of lymphedema; however, approximately 10% of all cases develop from primary lymphedema or situations where people are born with inadequate lymphatic systems. Other causes of lymphedema include radiation and trauma from motor vehicle accidents, falls, or other injuries to soft tissues.

Any time a surgery is performed on the body (not just after lymph node removal), lymphatics are disrupted. In these cases, only a very small disruption occurs and the lymphatic system easily accommodates this by using other pathways to transport fluid. However, scar tissue anywhere in the body may hamper lymphatic fluid flow. Remember that surgical incisions create scar tissue not only on the surface of the skin but down deep into the tissue. If this scar tissue is thick and prominent, it forms a barrier that the lymphatic vessels cannot move fluid through. In situations where there is significant scar tissue, there may be a swelling build-up, or lymphedema, surrounding the incision.

If you have an inherited condition that has malformed your lymphatic vessels, you may live for years and be unaware that your system is diminished. In this situation, your system is already functioning at a lower capacity and minor traumas such as sprains, burns, infections, or other local trauma will have a greater impact on overloading your system and can result in lymphedema. These situations trigger the onset of lymphedema in a previously healthy, nonswollen limb.

7. Is lymphedema painful?

Lymphedema is most commonly not a painful condition. The accumulation of lymphatic fluid in the tissue does not normally cause the pain sensors in the tissue to become aggravated. However, there are some areas of the body like the scrotum and the breast that contain

Lymphedema is most commonly not a painful condition.

exceptionally sensitive tissues. If lymphedema develops in these areas, it may be exceptionally painful.

Experiencing pain associated with lymphedema may be the result of other conditions. It is not unusual for the joints of the swollen limb to become painful over time—not because of the lymphedema, but because the limb is so large and heavy. When the joints are required to sustain this heavy load over a period of months or years, there may be pain that occurs from the overuse or degeneration of the joint. Further, if the size of the limb causes you to have to walk differently or adjust your posture to maneuver the limb, this strain may cause pain.

Pain can also be brought on by other, more emergent issues. An infection of the tissue will cause significant pain. Blood clots in the limb are also painful. Additionally, if a cancerous tumor is growing in an area where there is lymphedema, it may be pressing up against nerves and/or blocking blood flow from the limb and can cause substantial pain. Experiencing a new onset of pain in a limb with lymphedema should encourage follow-up with your doctor to ensure that one of these conditions is not causing your pain.

Red Flags

Red flags are changes that occur in the limb (or in your body) that should prompt you to seek medical attention. They may include:

- Redness on the limb that was not present before and seems to be worsening
- Redness associated with tissue that is warm or hot to the touch
- A new lump or thickening on the limb or in the region of the body affected with swelling

- A new, rapid onset of swelling
- A new onset of pain in the limb
- Fever, chills, and body aches
- Areas of the limb that seep or weep fluid with no apparent injury to the tissue

These conditions may be associated with several different conditions, including infections, blood clots, recurrent cancer, or new cancer tumors. Many times these situations come on quickly and can progress quickly. Every effort should be made to seek medical attention if you see these signs and symptoms.

Bonnie says:

Pain was the first clue that I had lymphedema. A couple of months after my mastectomy, the pain started in my chest. None of the pain meds I tried even took the edge off. It was hard for me to judge if there was swelling or not because I still wasn't used to the way my chest should look after the surgery. I'd heard of chest lymphedema, and since my doctors couldn't find any other cause for my pain, I found a well-trained lymphedema therapist who could diagnose and treat it. Once therapy started, I was amazed at how quickly the pain subsided. Now I only have pain when my lymphedema is out of control, so the pain helps motivate me to take good care of myself!

8. Can the swelling spread throughout my body?

Your lymphatic system is set up so that fluid from specific areas of the body is drained by specific parts of the lymphatic system. The general direction of fluid movement in the lymphatic system is from the furthest points away from the body (i.e., hands and feet) toward the central parts of the body. Each arm or leg has a specific pathway of lymph vessels that drains fluid to a specific basin of lymph nodes before it moves into the central lymphatic system. Because these pathways are specific to the region of the body, there is very little overlap of the vessels that drain fluid from the limbs. The trunk, abdomen, and head region vary a bit. These areas also have specific lymph vessels and nodes that drain fluid; however, there is more crossover between the vessels in these areas (**Figure 2**).

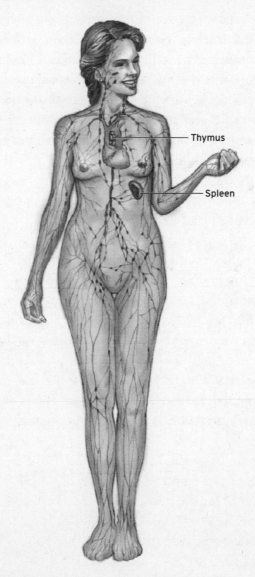

— Thymus

— Spleen

Figure 2   Lymphatic vessels.

Clark, Robert K. *Anatomy and Physiology: Understanding the Human Body, 2005; V-309.*

Lymphedema develops in a region of the body related to where the lymph nodes or vessels were damaged, very much like a traffic jam that occurs on the highways near an accident.

Lymphedema develops in a region of the body related to where the lymph nodes or vessels were damaged, very much like a traffic jam that occurs on the highways near an accident. We can imagine that a substantial traffic accident on a major highway will cause traffic to back up. The back-up occurs not only on the highway but also on the ramps leading to the highway; if the traffic sits long enough, it can even back up onto the surrounding neighborhood roads. The back-up occurs along the roads leading to the accident—that is, if there is another major highway a few miles away with no traffic accident, you would not see the traffic back up onto this highway too. The lymphatic system works much like this description of traffic; the vessels that drain one arm are a good distance away from those that drain the other arm, and a back-up in one will not typically affect the other.

There are, however, places where the major highways of the lymphatic system come together and a large amount of fluid "traffic" is merging. If there is an injury to the lymphatic system here, then the region that congests with fluid might involve more areas of the body. For example, in the abdomen there are several large lymph vessels that bring fluid up from the legs and merge together. If there is damage near the place where they merge, then there is a risk for both legs to swell.

When there has been known damage to the lymphatic system, such as lymph nodes being removed from the armpit, groin, or the neck, we can be fairly certain that swelling related to this damage will not spread to other areas of the body. If the swelling is related to a hereditary condition and we are not sure where, or how much of, the system is damaged, there may be swelling in several different body regions.

9. Can lymphedema run in my family?

Yes. As discussed in Question 4, about 10% of the lymphedema in the United States is hereditary and is called primary lymphedema. If the lymphedema is present at birth, it is called congenital and is most likely inherited lymphedema. When it occurs later in life, it can be more difficult to determine if the lymphedema is hereditary or has some other cause. In this instance, it is important to survey the family history for family members with lymphedema. The age of onset can be helpful in determining which kind of lymphedema is present.

Hereditary lymphedema may present differently from one generation to the next and may even skip a generation in its presentation. If the condition presents in each generation of the family, it is called familial and is associated with an autosomal dominant trait. When the condition skips a generation, it is called sporadic. Sporadic conditions are associated with a genetic trait that is weaker, or recessive. Even if the condition is sporadic in its presentation, the generation that does not have the condition still carries the gene and may pass it on to the next generation. Therefore, it is important to recognize other members of your family who have lymphedema and to understand the type of lymphedema they have. A genetic form of lymphedema in your blood relative may put you at risk for eventually developing lymphedema and of passing that trait on to your children.

Bonnie says:

My bilateral arm and chest lymphedema showed up following mastectomies for breast cancer, but only one node was removed from the cancerous side, and on the other side no nodes were purposely removed or damaged. With such a low risk for lymphedema I wondered how I could have developed it. I figured maybe I was just more susceptible to lymphedema because of a genetic predisposition, so I started researching my family's medical history. I didn't find any evidence of lymphedema in my relatives, but I did discover other words for lymphedema that were used in earlier days, like "dropsy" and "milk leg." If you're asking older relatives about your family's history of lymphedema, you might find out more if you use these older words to describe it.

10. How do I get lymphedema treated or cured?

Currently, there is no cure for lymphedema. Techniques for treating the condition exist and are effective to a large degree to decrease the overall size of the limb and to maintain the limb size; however, the condition will never go away completely due to the body's inability to regrow new lymphatic vessels and nodes once they have been damaged or surgically removed.

Lymphedema is different from other types of edema because it is its own disease. Many other types of swelling exist in the body and are signs or symptoms of another condition or disease state. Lymphedema is itself the disease state and perpetuates its own development in the body.

Many different types of treatment strategies will be discussed in later sections of this book. They are designed to help prevent the onset of lymphedema, prevent or arrest the progression of lymphedema, and decongest the swollen limb. These techniques are very effective but will not permanently cure the condition.

11. What if I don't treat the lymphedema?

Untreated lymphedema is very likely to worsen. Patients with mild lymphedema (stage 1) often can do with only very minimal treatment to control their swelling. However, if mild lymphedema is not treated appropriately, protein will gradually build up in the tissue and can develop into a more pronounced swelling (**Figure 3**). Patients with stage 2 or 3 lymphedema will need to do daily self-care, as prescribed by their medical team; otherwise, over time the limb(s) will increase in size. **Table 1** describes the symptoms related to each stage of lymphedema.

Along with the larger size of the limb, there are changes that take place in the tissue of the limb

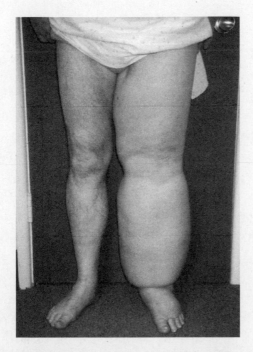

Figure 3   Stage II Lymphedema; abnormal contour is noted throughout the limb.

The Basics

Table 1   Staging of Lymphedema (Based on the International Society of Lymphology)

STAGE 0: Latency	• Lymph nodes and vessels have been removed and/or damaged • No visible swelling exists • Sensory changes may occur
STAGE I	• Visible edema exists in the limb and is usually pitting • The swelling may exacerbate and remit • Elevation of the limb helps to reduce the swelling
STAGE II	• Swelling does not spontaneously reverse with elevation or rest • Fibrosis (scarring) is evident in the tissue • The edema may or may not be pitting
STAGE III	• Marked swelling of the limb • Hardened tissue • Skin becomes rough and thickened • Oozing and weeping of fluid may be seen

when lymphedema is untreated. These changes result in scarring and lead to fibrosis, a more advanced condition that requires more intensive treatment. Fibrosis will cause the limb to feel firmer over time and eventually to become very hard. This scarring of the tissue further damages the remaining healthy vessels and contributes to even greater swelling. The texture of the skin may also change as lymphedema goes untreated. The skin becomes rough and thickened, much like that of an elephant. In the very advanced stages, lymphedema is called **elephantiasis** because of these skin changes. The hardened skin is dry and is likely to crack and chafe, leading to open areas on the limb that may weep fluid and serve as entry points for bacteria that may cause lethal infections.

Elephantiasis

A condition of the skin whereby there is thickening and multiple layers of skin form on top of one another. The skin takes on a scaly appearance and is very rough and thick.

When lymphedema is untreated, the congestion in the tissue is rich with protein and can serve as an excellent medium for bacteria to thrive. Also, because the lymphatic system is working less effectively, there is a higher risk for infection. Untreated lymphedema may lead to frequent dangerous infections.

In very rare circumstances, a condition called lymphangiosarcoma may arise if lymphedema is left untreated in an advanced stage. This is a **malignant** tumor that grows in the soft tissue resulting from the long-standing nature of the untreated lymphedema. The condition is often deadly at this point. Lymphangiosarcoma is a rare condition that can occur in untreated, uncontrolled lymphedema.

Do not worry if you miss a day or two of your prescribed treatment, but do not make it a habit. Over time, you have learned about your limb and you know how it will best respond under certain circumstances. You likely have also learned how far you can push the limits before you will see a negative effect of not treating it appropriately. If you do experience an increase in your swelling, your medical team will work with you to bring the condition back under control.

Untreated lymphedema may lead to frequent dangerous infections.

Malignant
(1) A condition that tends to be severe and become progressively worse.
(2) In regard to a tumor, having the ability to invade and destroy nearby tissue and spread (metastasize) to other parts of the body.

Bonnie says:

I have friends with lymphedema who don't treat it. It's a choice we all have to make ourselves. Their limbs are hard now, their clothes have to be altered by a seamstress to fit them, and sometimes their skin oozes lymph fluid. Treating lymphedema takes time and it can be discouraging, so I understand the choice they've made. But for myself, the extra work and effort pay off in peace of mind, good control of the swelling, and lower infection risk.

12. Are there doctors who specialize in lymphedema?

Yes, but there are very few here in the United States. The lymphatic system structure and function is not a significant part of the current medical school curriculum, so there are only few physicians in the United States who have both knowledge and an interest in lymphatic disorders. Most of these physicians specialize in rehabilitation medicine and have focused experience in diagnosing and managing lymphedema. Additionally, doctors who are vascular specialists have a better understanding of the lymphatic system and its disorders.

13. What medical providers can I see for the treatment of lymphedema?

Over the last decade, hundreds of clinicians in the United States have been taught the specialized techniques for managing lymphedema. The majority of the clinicians are physical and occupational therapists. Nurses and massage therapists also work in this field. Most therapists who treat lymphedema work in clinics affiliated with a major medical center or a hospital-based outpatient center. However, it is becoming more common to see smaller community hospitals and clinics offering comprehensive lymphedema treatment. There are also therapists and nurses who may be able to come to your home to treat lymphedema.

Therapists who treat lymphedema should have a level of specialized training, which they have achieved by taking specialty courses. Many of these specialists go on to be certified by the Lymphology Association of North America (LANA). This means they have taken a specific amount of course work in lymphedema and have passed a national examination.

Optimally, your medical team should consist of a physician who you see regularly to ensure that the condition is well controlled. You should also have a therapist who is a specialist in lymphedema management as a part of your medical team. This is the person who will work with you to not only treat the condition and decongest the limb but also teach you how to maintain the condition over time. A close collaboration between you and your medical team is vital to ensure that your condition is managed optimally.

Jan says:

When I first discovered I had arm lymphedema, the breast surgeon who made the diagnosis referred me to a team of lymphedema therapists in a hospital-based outpatient center. When my hand swelled up several years later, my oncologist referred me to a lymphedema therapist with her own independent practice. She was not affiliated with a hospital or a clinic. Being LANA-certified, all these therapists were effective in reducing general and stubborn swelling using CDT (complete decongestive therapy).

14. Where can I locate a clinic to be treated?

Many specialty health care teams and clinics are affiliated with hospitals and large outpatient-based therapy clinics. The National Lymphedema Network (NLN) provides a list of therapists and specialty clinics around the country. You can find their listing on the NLN Web site (www.lymphnet.org) or in *LymphLink*, the official NLN quarterly newsletter. You can also call your local hospital or outpatient rehabilitation clinic and ask if they have a lymphedema program or a lymphedema specialist on staff. Your insurance company may also be able to give you a list of therapists who treat lymphedema and are covered by your insurance plan.

The Appendix at the end of this book offers a number of Web sites that you can use to search for help. Also, there are many schools that give educational courses in lymphedema treatment, and they often will list their graduates on their Web page. This serves as an additional resource for you to seek out therapists who have received specialty education. If you have not yet been diagnosed with lymphedema but believe you are experiencing symptoms of this condition, see Question 33 for information on finding a specialist to make the correct diagnosis.

PART TWO

Risk Factors for Lymphedema

If I have lymph nodes taken out, what is my risk for developing lymphedema?

Are there exercises and activities I should avoid that may cause lymphedema?

Is it true that tight clothing could cause lymphedema?

More . . .

A Note about Risk Factors and "Risk Reduction"

This section of the book focuses on practices aimed at reducing risk for the person who does NOT have lymphedema but who may be predisposed or "at risk" because he or she has had lymph nodes removed or has had other therapies that have damaged the lymphatic system. It is difficult to talk about the concept of "prevention" of lymphedema because we have no absolute way of preventing lymphedema once the system has been damaged. The authors hope to offer guidelines, based on evidence where applicable and on sound physiological principles, that will help to reduce the risk of developing lymphedema.

15. If I have lymph nodes taken out, what is my risk for developing lymphedema?

There are patients who have had dozens of lymph nodes removed and never developed lymphedema. Then there are patients who have only one or two nodes removed, and they develop lymphedema soon after their surgery and/or radiation therapy. We do not know the structure and anatomy of each individual's lymphatic system prior to surgery, but many people may be born with a compromised lymphatic system that never causes any swelling until they have a minor surgery or trauma. When these people are exposed to lymph node and vessel damage, despite following strict risk-reduction practices, they may develop lymphedema.

Having lymph nodes taken out does not mean that you will absolutely develop lymphedema. The overall risk of developing lymphedema after surgery to remove lymph nodes ranges from 4 to 30%, depending on the number of nodes taken out and other treatments delivered, such as radiation therapy. The lowest risk is associated with the sentinel lymph node biopsy (SLNB); if this is the surgery conducted, the risk of developing lymphedema is reported to range from 4 to 8%. When an SLNB is performed followed by radiation therapy, that risk reportedly doubles to approximately 16%. If an axillary lymph node dissection (ALND) is the surgery performed, the risk for lymphedema ranges from 12 to 17%; when radiation therapy is given in addition, the risk again doubles and is reported to be from 30 to 45%. Melanoma surgeries also carry a risk of developing lymphedema, with incidence rates ranging from 17 to 45%.

It is important to understand what lymphedema is and to recognize the symptoms that might tell you if you are developing lymphedema. Your risk is higher if you have had a greater number of lymph nodes removed, if you have had radiation therapy, and if you have gained weight since your initial treatment.

16. What if my surgery was several years ago? Am I still at risk?

Patients who have had surgeries specifically to remove lymph nodes from the armpit, the groin, or the neck area will be at risk of developing lymphedema for the rest of their lives. This ongoing risk is because the lymphatic system is unable to grow new vessels and nodes to replace those that were taken. However, the further away from the surgery you are, the less chance there is of developing lymphedema. Over time, your body learns to use lymphatic vessels that are still healthy to help make up for the ones that were taken. Once these alternate pathways are established, the body can handle the fluid in a more efficient manner and there may be a lower risk of swelling. The first few years after a surgery, your body is finding and learning ways to use these alternate pathways.

Risk Factors for Lymphedema

Your risk of developing lymphedema is higher if you have had a greater number of lymph nodes removed, if you have had radiation therapy, and if you have gained weight since your initial treatment.

Practicing risk reduction is important for anyone who has had lymph nodes removed. Although the risk decreases over time, it still exists, and diligent attention must be paid to the limb to protect it from infections and other potentially harmful triggers.

17. Will air travel cause lymphedema?

The air pressure around us is supportive of our skin and our blood vessels. It gently pushes against us to support our vessels and prevents too much fluid from escaping into the tissue. During a flight, the air pressure in the airplane decreases from the normal pressure we are used to on the ground to a much lower pressure at a high altitude. The decreased pressure within the plane's cabin applies less of a force against our skin and allows more fluid to escape into the tissue.

All of the fluid that ends up in the body's tissue must be absorbed and transported away by the lymphatic system to prevent swelling. If too much fluid gets into the tissue, the damaged system has difficulty keeping up and there may be swelling. If the lymphatic system is damaged from a prior surgery or trauma, the increased fluid in the body tissues has even more of a negative effect because it is much harder for the damaged system to remove that excess fluid. Flying in a plane for a period of time can cause swelling even when none had existed before. It can also worsen existing lymphedema unless appropriate compression is applied to the limb. (Compression is discussed extensively in Part 4.)

Individuals who have had surgery to remove lymph nodes have difficulty absorbing excess fluids that escape in the tissues. If you have had lymph nodes removed, you are considered to be "at risk" and should pay close attention to changes in sensations of the extremities (i.e., heaviness, fullness, or aching), as these may be early signs of swelling in the tissue.

People who have lymphedema are at a greater risk of having the condition worsen on an airplane flight if they do not wear compression on their limb. If we introduce more fluid to the tissue, we are further burdening an already dysfunctional system and the swelling may get worse.

It is important to remember that there are many factors that may bring about swelling in the limb on a travel day, including:

- **Dehydration**: Remember to hydrate well and avoid alcohol, especially during long flights, as dehydration may further increase the risk of swelling.
- **Immobility**: Move around the cabin frequently and stretch to keep the muscles and joints moving, thereby allowing greater movement of fluid out of the tissues.
- **Overuse of the extremity**: If possible, carry luggage on wheels and refrain from carrying heavy purses and large shoulder bags, as this can be very straining and harmful to the limb. Remember to allow plenty of time to get through airports. Extended periods of high exertion may tax the lymphatic system, as more and more blood flow and lymphatic fluid must be processed.

Important: Patients who are "at risk" should consider wearing a correctly fitted garment (sleeve/stocking) on a flight to prevent the onset of lymphedema. The garment should be worn for several hours prior to the flight to ensure that it is not too loose or too tight. The garment should be prescribed and fitted by your medical team to ensure that it is appropriate for you (see Question 39).

Bonnie says:

The lymphedema in my right arm started on a plane trip from Phoenix to a small town in Alaska. By the time I arrived, my hand had swollen up like a baseball mitt. It was painful and frightening, and of course there was no one in that little town who could help me. The trip home was even more frightening, since I knew it would swell again—and it did! Once I got back to my own medical team, I was able to get help quickly. A well-fitted sleeve and glove would have been a big help and assurance in that situation when I was so far from home.

Jan says:

After my axillary node dissection, I flew several times for business on flights lasting 10–11 hours. Before I took these flights, the doctors did not warn me that I should be fitted for and wear a compression sleeve to reduce my risk of developing lymphedema. In addition, I did not move around the cabin frequently, nor did I drink adequate water. Shortly after one of these flights, when I sustained a garden injury on my affected arm, I noticed swelling that developed into lymphedema.

18. If I have had lymph nodes removed, should I avoid blood pressures being taken on that arm?

Although insufficient research has been done regarding blood pressure measures, you should be cautious about having your blood pressure taken on the limb where lymph nodes were removed. If your medical provider is taking the blood pressure measurement by hand, and does so correctly, the risk for developing lymphedema is likely to be low. However, the pneumatic, automatic blood pressure pumps that are commonly used today present more of a risk, as they may exert excessive pressure on the limb and damage delicate lymphatic vessels. In situations where an automatic blood pressure cuff is used repeatedly for a long period of time, such as during surgery or during polygraph testing, the at-risk limb should not be used.

Making every effort to have blood pressure taken on the opposite side from the site of your surgery is the safest option. For some people who have bilateral removal of axillary lymph nodes, there is a way that blood pressure can be taken on the leg with equal accuracy. This will require your medical provider to use a larger-sized blood pressure cuff that will be applied to the top of the leg. Although the technique is different, it can be done with great accuracy.

If you are in a medical emergency, your blood pressure might need to be taken from the affected arm. Wearing a lymphedema alert bracelet will alert paramedics, physicians in the ER, or lab technicians to refrain from taking blood pressure in the affected area. *Despite the many anecdotes of patients developing lymphedema from having their blood pressure taken, we have no science to support this as a risk factor.*

19. Are there exercises and activities I should avoid that may cause lymphedema?

Exercise is an integral part of a healthy lifestyle. It is important for patients with or at risk for lymphedema to understand that they can safely perform aerobic and resistive exercises using the affected body part(s) when:

1. They consult with their medical team for guidance with their exercise program.
2. The "at-risk" limb is not exercised to fatigue.
3. Trauma and overuse is prevented.

Despite the many anecdotes of patients developing lymphedema from having their blood pressure taken, we have no science to support this as a risk factor.

Each individual is different, and it is important to initiate exercise at a low intensity, gradually increasing the repetitions and weights. Types of exercise include:

- **Flexibility and stretching exercises**: These exercises are recommended to support muscle and connective tissue, minimize scarring, and enhance lymph flow.
- **Resistive exercise**: This type of exercise has been formally studied and shown to enhance lymph flow and prevent limb swelling from muscle overuse. Monitor the limb closely, as strength training can increase local blood flow and potentially trigger or worsen existing lymphedema.
- **Aerobic exercise**: Such exercise can include walking, jogging, cycling, and swimming. It is performed continuously using large muscle groups and requires 60–75% of the individual maximum heart rate. Aerobics enhance the cardiovascular fitness, weight management, and venous/lymphatic flow—as well as overall outlook on life.

Jan says:

I make it my routine to visit our local fitness club at least three times weekly. During each of these workouts, I perform aerobic exercise for at least 30 minutes. I prefer the arc trainer, step machine, and treadmill to keep aerobically fit, since the exercises on these machines strengthen the bones to avoid osteoporosis, a debilitating disease that poses a special risk for cancer patients. On two of these weekly jaunts, I perform resistive exercise, lifting free weights up to 7 pounds and engaging in chin-up and pull-down exercises, using appropriately light weight on a Gravitron machine. I do many heavy-duty leg resistive exercises since my legs have no swelling. In addition, using an exercise ball, I perform active elongation stretches learned from my lymphedema therapist to stretch my scars.

And I make sure to stretch my calves and thighs before the aerobic phase to avoid injuries. Sometimes I also swim in the indoor pool at the club or participate in their aerobic swim classes.

20. Will needlesticks cause lymphedema?

Patients who are "at risk" have had their lymphatic system altered, and their capacity to handle fluid will always be compromised. Protecting the skin integrity is of the utmost importance to reduce the risk of developing an infection and/or creating an inflammatory process that may bring on a bout of swelling and cause lymphedema where none had existed before. If possible, effort should be made to avoid injections or the placement of intravenous (IV) lines in the affected limb.

Any time the skin integrity is damaged, there is a risk that bacteria may enter the tissue and promote an infection. This risk is heightened for those who have had lymph nodes removed. A single injection to the tissue carries a relatively low risk; however, because of the needle puncture, there is a risk. A greater risk exists when an IV is placed into the limb. An IV is a line placed into the vein that enables blood to be drawn or medications to be delivered to the body. When an IV line is placed, there is a more prolonged inflammatory response to this indwelling needle than there is with just a single needle puncture. In addition, when an IV line is placed, many times it stays inside the vein for several days. These factors increase the risk of allowing bacteria into the tissue and causing an infection.

Another consideration is for patients who are diabetic and are required to closely monitor their blood glucose levels by doing needlesticks to their fingers to obtain blood samples. Such repeated needlesticks have been shown to correlate to a greater risk of developing lymphedema.

There are many anecdotes of patients developing lymphedema shortly after a needlestick or IV placement. There is research to support that skin punctures such as these correlate to the development of lymphedema. It is advisable to encourage your healthcare provider to avoid needles in the affected arm(s) or leg(s) to reduce the risk.

Bonnie says:

It can be hard to convince healthcare providers to leave an at-risk arm alone. The National Lymphedema Network has a position paper on risk reduction practices (www.lymphnet. org) that you can bring with you to share with your doctor, nurse, or phlebotomist. It's your arm, so it's up to you to be calm but firm about insisting that your at-risk arm not be used for blood tests, injections, or IVs.

21. Does extreme heat or cold cause lymphedema?

Extreme heat often causes swelling in many people, but patients who have had node dissection and/or have a known insufficiency of their lymphatic system are especially at risk of developing lymphedema with prolonged exposure to heat.

Important: During warm summer months, make sure to cover the affected arm(s) or leg(s) with a loose cotton sleeve or slacks and avoid direct sunlight. Also use sunscreen when swimming and avoid sunburn. Effort should also be taken to avoid applying hot packs or heating pads directly to the at-risk areas of the body. The application of heat causes an increase in blood flow to the body region. If the region has insufficiency in the lymphatic system, it will be difficult to manage the fluid load associated with the increased blood flow, and swelling may result.

Cold exposure also causes a constriction of the lymph vessels and may render them less effective when the exposure is extreme or prolonged. When the vessels are not working correctly, there is a chance that swelling may occur and cause a new onset of lymphedema where none had previously existed.

22. Is it true that tight clothing could cause lymphedema?

It is prudent to forgo tight clothing that may form a tourniquet-like structure on the limb. It is reasonable to believe that a tourniquet around the limb may cause swelling by compromising the outflow of blood and lymph. If we translate this to clothing, it is advisable to avoid clothing with tight waistbands, socks, tight sleeves, and even bra bands and straps that are too tight.

The concern with tight clothing is the restriction it places on the very small lymph vessels located just under the skin. These lymphatic vessels are important for collecting and moving lymph fluid through its cycle of circulation. If these vessels are blocked, there is a chance that a back-up could occur.

There is no research to support the correlation of tight clothing with the onset of lymphedema, but if we use our common sense, we can deduce that any clothing that puts undue pressure on the limb and even restricts blood flow may be harmful in someone who has a compromised lymphatic system. Therefore, avoiding clothing that constricts the tissue to the degree of

Any clothing that puts undue pressure on the limb and even restricts blood flow may be harmful in someone who has a compromised lymphatic system.

37

causing skin redness may potentially minimize the risk of developing lymphedema.

23. Is it true that cutting my nails can cause lymphedema?

It is the not actual cutting the nail that may contribute to the development of lymphedema. However, when the nails and cuticles are cut, there is a risk that the skin may be damaged and potentially introduce bacteria into the tissue.

We carry bacteria on our skin all the time, and our hands (and feet) are exposed to more bacteria than many other areas of our body. When we suffer a small cut from a cuticle tear, there is a risk that the normal bacteria we encounter with our hands may become harmful and introduce an infection into our tissue. As the body fights infection, inflammation occurs. If the lymphatic system has been damaged, even in the absence of lymphedema, the infection and inflammation can cause swelling in the tissue; if the lymphatic system is not able to carry the fluid away after the infection, lymphedema may result. It is advisable to avoid open areas on our skin, such as a cuticle cut, thorns from the garden, insect bites, or cat scratches, as this may increase the risk of an infection.

Jan says:

If I have hangnails, I cut them carefully. To prevent cracks around my nails, I apply an ample quantity of skin cream to my hands, especially in winter when the inside air is so dry. Also, instead of getting acrylic nails, I use fingernail polish, since I understand that the technique for getting acrylic nails may cause infection. Sally Hansen's clear Hard As Nails fingernail polish works best for me. If you want to indulge in a manicure, bring your own tools rather than risk an infection from nonsterile tools.

PART THREE

Diagnosis and Differential Diagnosis

About the early signs and symptoms of lymphedema—are there warning signs?

How do I know if I just have swelling or if it is lymphedema?

What tests should I have done to diagnose lymphedema?

More . . .

24. About the early signs and symptoms of lymphedema—are there warning signs?

In the case of primary lymphedema, the first concern for possible development of lymphedema would be a positive family history. There is a high transmittal of hereditary and congenital types of lymphedema— approximately a 50% transmission rate from one generation to the next. Females are more at risk of inheriting primary lymphedema. Typically, the early signs include intermittent swelling of the distal limb, most often seen in the feet or the ankles, which will resolve with elevation of the limb. This swelling can occur more obviously when the temperatures are very high, with prolonged standing, or around the time of the menstrual cycle. In the early stages, the swelling may exacerbate and remit and even appear to go away for a period of time. However, these repeated instances of mild swelling will contribute to a slow congestion of protein in the body tissue. Over time, the edema may not resolve as well with just elevating the legs and eventually will remain in the tissue for more prolonged periods of time.

In secondary lymphedema, there are also early signs and symptoms of onset. Some people are at greater risk than others and should pay close attention if they notice early signs of change in the limb. Remember that once lymph nodes are removed or damaged, there is a lifelong risk for that person to develop lymphedema. It is important for those people to be familiar with the risk reductions that are recommended by the National Lymphedema Network (NLN) (www.lymphnet.org).

Often, individuals will report that their lymphedema occurred shortly after suffering an infection following surgical intervention. Research has shown that people who have experienced a postoperative infection at the surgical site may be at a greater risk for developing lymphedema. Other factors associated with the onset of lymphedema include seroma formation (the pocketing of fluid at the incision site after surgery), greater number of lymph nodes removed, radiation therapy, and increased body weight. If you meet these risk factors, it is important to know the early signs and symptoms that occur with lymphedema.

Some of the initial changes in the limb are detected by sensory observations. People will note that they experience a tight, full feeling. Other descriptions of sensory changes include a tingly feeling in the affected limb, heaviness, and aching. Other common early signs of lymphedema include a visible swelling of the hand or around the joints of the wrist and/or elbow. These are important signs to note and address with your medical provider. In these early instances, the swelling may visibly seem to go away completely. However, there are still changes that have occurred in the tissue that warrant attention from your specialist.

If an intervention can be introduced at this early stage, the progress of the swelling may be prevented. Even if the swelling seems to go away or appears to be very mild, it is still important to seek treatment to prevent the condition from progressing to an advanced stage.

25. What if there is only a little bit of swelling in my limb? Should I do anything about it?

If the limb has been exposed to radiation, surgery, or any other trauma, it is very important to be observant of changes in the limb and to act upon them. Many people experience transient swelling because of excessive salt and water intake, exposure to heat, and/or sitting for prolonged periods of time with their feet hanging down. Also, some medications cause mild generalized swelling. In these situations, the swelling will tend to be system-wide, instead of localized to only one area. When the swelling is confined to the limb or body region where the system has been damaged, there is a higher level of concern than if there is generalized swelling that affects many body regions.

If swelling occurs only in the limb or body region associated with the damaged lymphatics, even if only a small amount of swelling exists, it should be evaluated by your medical team (**Figure 4**). When this type of swelling occurs, it is important to unload the demands on the lymphatic system as much as possible. This may be

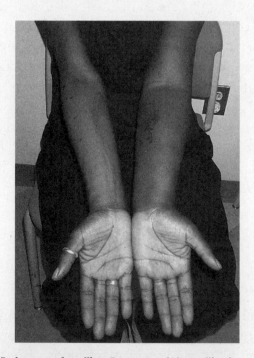

Figure 4   **Early onset of swelling. Even very subtle swelling in the limb should be addressed by your medical provider.**

achieved by elevating the affected limb, applying light compression (if directed by your medical team) to encourage reduction of fluid, and/or improving mobility of the body region to help restore more normal lymphatic function.

Even a very small amount of swelling in the affected limb can be problematic if not adequately managed. The nature of lymphedema is to progress gradually over time when it is not appropriately cared for. If you are able to seek medical care as soon as the swelling occurs, you may be able to halt the progression of the swelling and keep it very well controlled.

26. What if the swelling is only in the chest or the abdomen? Is this still lymphedema?

Lymphedema can occur in any part of the body, not just arms and legs. It can occur in the face, neck, chest, breast, and genitals, and it can be very difficult to treat in these locations. Lymphatics are present in all parts of the body that are covered with skin; thus, lymphedema can occur anywhere in the body. If swelling occurs in a body region where lymphatics have been damaged, the resultant swelling is lymphedema.

Breast lymphedema, sometimes seen after breast conservation surgeries and radiation therapy, can be very problematic. Lymphedema may also occur in the chest wall, the back, and even in the armpit after treatment of breast cancer. Especially difficult are genital lymphedema and abdominal lymphedema.

Treating lymphedema in these body regions is challenging. Not only are the contours of these body regions difficult to apply compression to, but these tissues do not have a substantial amount of muscle tissue.

Lymphatics are present in all parts of the body that are covered with skin; thus, lymphedema can occur anywhere in the body.

The muscle pumping action is an important component of fluid evacuation with short-stretch bandages. The bandages are most effective when the large muscle groups are working, as the counterpressure from the bandages effectively evacuates fluid. The truncal body regions do not have large, bulky muscle groups, making the compression strategies more challenging. Compression that accommodates the body contours without causing areas of constriction will be most effective to reduce the edema. Optimal decongestion will be achieved with consistent compression applied to the tissue over time as part of a comprehensive decongestive therapy program.

Bonnie says:

My chest was the first place that lymphedema appeared. It was hard to find a health professional to diagnose it and send me to the right therapist for treatment because many of them are only familiar with lymphedema in the limbs. All that effort to get a diagnosis made me feel like it must be all in my head. So it was reassuring, when I finally had my first appointment with a knowledgeable lymphedema therapist, to hear her say, "You have lymphedema in your chest, and we're going to do something about it."

27. If my legs are swollen, is there a risk I may get swelling in my abdomen or genitals?

Yes, there is a risk. Very often, inguinal, pelvic, or abdominal lymph nodes are involved in the onset of lymphedema occurring in a leg. Lymphatic fluid from the genital regions must also travel to these lymph nodes. Since fluid from the genitals moves along many of the same pathways as fluid from the legs, all of this fluid must have a clear pathway or congestion may occur at any point. Therefore, injury to these lymph nodes will commonly affect the legs and may result in genital and/or scrotal lymphedema.

Optimal decongestive treatment of the lower extremities should not cause swelling of the genitals. Pneumatic pump devices are effective at treating leg lymphedema, however, if they are used on the leg without proper treatment of the lymphatic system, there is a risk that genital swelling may occur. Utilizing correct manual lymph drainage (MLD) techniques and compression strategies at the genital region when utilizing a compression pump will help to reduce this risk.

28. Will genital or scrotal edema make me impotent or infertile?

If left untreated, very advanced lymphedema of the genitals and scrotum can result in erectile dysfunction due to fibrosis and scarring of the phallus; eventually, without treatment, moderate to severe scrotal edema can result in impotence. This condition is due in part to the inability of the scrotum to control the temperature of the testes. Because thickened fibrotic or fluid-filled skin covers the testes, they will remain at too high a temperature, and the sperm will no longer be potent.

29. If lymph nodes were removed from my neck, can I get swelling in my face and neck?

Face and neck lymphedema may occur after the treatment for head and neck cancers (**Figure 5**). Removal of a single lymph node rarely results in swelling of the face and neck because so many alternate paths and lymph nodes are available in this region. However, with radical dissections in which a large number of lymph nodes and significant amount of tissue are removed from the neck area, lymphedema can occur. The risk increases markedly with the addition of radiation therapy. Swelling may

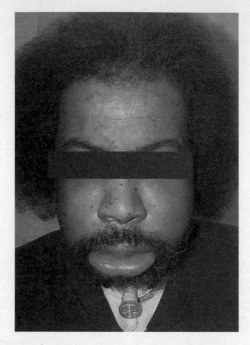

Figure 5   Facial lymphedema, following surgery for a cancer of the neck.

occur anywhere in the facial region, including the mouth, ears, neck, scalp and eyes.

Treating head and neck lymphedema can be very successful. Finding alternate drainage paths usually through the posterior head and neck area is important in the manual drainage treatment, and compression garments can be fabricated for comfortable wear. During the day, when a person is standing and moving, the swelling may seem to decrease because gravity is assisting the drainage of the face and neck. Compression garments are difficult to wear during the daytime hours, as they may be cumbersome and limit speech, sight, and overall head mobility. However, at times of rest and especially at night, achieving consistent compression application is important.

30. How do I know if I just have swelling or if it is lymphedema?

Most often lymphedema is recognized because it can be associated with specific events—for example, surgery with lymph node removal, radiation therapy, or family history of lymphedema occurring in close relatives. If the edema occurs without an obvious cause, it is important to make sure that other causes have been eliminated. Edema may often occur with **congestive heart failure** or can be seen in patients with renal failure. It is also present in patients with hormonal changes at the time of their menses. Edema can also be seen with other conditions, such as allergic reaction, inflammatory arthritis, or venous abnormalities.

If other medical conditions have been ruled out and there is no obvious cause of the edema, then it is important to have a physical examination by a lymphedema specialist. Often, through a simple clinical examination, a specialist can give you an accurate diagnosis and assist you in finding appropriate treatment. A specific diagnostic test, called a lymphoscintigraphy may be recommended. This test measures the function of the lymphatic system in a limb. The test involves a radioactive substance that is injected into the limb and measured to determine how it moves through the limb over time in comparison to a normal limb. If there are abnormalities in the lymphatic transport of the substance, then the abnormality of the lymphatic system can be diagnosed. This test does not identify the cause of the lymphedema but helps to rule out edema from other non-lymphatic causes.

There are specific signs and symptoms associated with the presentation of lymphedema that your medical provider will be able to identify in making the correct diagnosis. Lymphedema tends to occur most often in a

Congestive heart failure

An abnormal condition of impaired cardiac pumping, due to heart muscle tissue that has been injured.

limb, more frequently the lower extremities if it is primary lymphedema. In secondary lymphedema, it will be associated with the body region where lymph nodes were damaged. Lymphedema is unique in that it will always present in an asymmetrical fashion. Even if both limbs are affected, one will be larger than the other if the swelling is due to a lymphatic disruption. Even when the diagnosis of lymphedema seems to be straightforward, it is important to consult with your healthcare provider to ensure that the correct diagnosis is made and that there are no additional medical problems contributing to the condition.

31. Sometimes the color of my limb changes. What does this mean?

When the limb changes colors, it is usually due to a change in the blood flow. Determining why the change occurred depends on the color to which the limb changes. A scarlet red or brilliant pink color is most often associated with cellulitis, which is an infection of the subcutaneous tissue (see Question 69). This condition is also sometimes referred to as **erysipelas** and is accompanied by skin that is warm to the touch and possibly by pain and a fever.

Erysipelas
An infectious skin disease characterized by redness, swelling, vesicles, fever, pain, and lymphade-nopathy. It is caused by a species of group A streptococci.

If the limb has a normal color when elevated, or propped up, and develops a deep, dark color when hanging down, this may indicate venous insufficiency. When the venous system cannot efficiently return blood from the distant areas of the body (usually the feet and lower legs), a blue or purple discoloration may persist over time and may be associated with swelling. The treatment for venous insufficiency requires the application of compression garments to the leg to help prevent venous congestion and promote better blood flow out of the limb.

If blood flow into the limb is diminished, this is usually because the arteries carrying blood are insufficient. This insufficiency usually results in a color change in which the limb is blanched or white. In this instance, the limb may also be painful with prolonged standing or walking, as there is not adequate blood flow to the tissue.

It is not unusual for a lymphedematous limb to have a persistent pinkish blush to the skin due to inflammation from the lymphedema itself. The presence of protein in the lymphedema within the interstitium can lead to a reactive inflammatory response with mild redness and very mild warmth even though there is no infection. Because the tissue is not infected, antibiotic treatment is not warranted. The best treatment is excellent management of the lymphedema to decongest the limb and maintain the swelling. This treatment will result in an overall decrease in inflammation and diminish the redness of the skin.

32. What tests should I have done to diagnose lymphedema?

Any time lymphedema is suspected, dangerous look-alikes should be ruled out immediately. The first and most important test should be for a **deep vein thrombosis (DVT)**. A DVT is a blood clot that is lodged in the vein and blocks the blood flow through the vein. This condition results in a back-up of blood into the limb with eventual redness, swelling, and pain. A **Doppler ultrasound study** can be used to detect DVTs in a limb, if pelvic clots are anticipated; a **spiral computed tomography (CT) scan** is the most sensitive test. If a Doppler or a CT study is negative for DVT, then having a **lymphoscintigraphy** with an experienced radiologist is the most reliable diagnostic test for lymphedema. **Magnetic resonance imaging**

Deep vein thrombosis (DVT)

A blood clot in one or more of the deep veins in the legs (most common), arms, pelvis, neck axilla, or chest.

Doppler ultrasound

A form of ultrasound that can detect blood flow. Commonly used to visualize blood obstructions to blood flow such as blood clots.

Spiral computed tomography (CT) scan

A technique that is performed by moving the patient continuously through the scanner and produces a more rapid and detailed scan of internal structures.

Lymphoscintigraphy
A method used to image the lymphatic vessels and nodes.

Magnetic resonance imaging

The production of cross sectional images by placing a body part in a static strong magnetic field and analyzing the resonance of hydrogen in various tissues.

(MRI) can be useful to identify swelling in the tissue, but it is not specific enough to diagnose lymphedema. In Europe, micro-lymphatic **angiography** is routinely performed to diagnose lymphedema when a genetic cause of lymphedema is suspected. This technique is not utilized routinely in the United States.

Once diagnostic tests have been done to rule out other conditions, an accurate clinical diagnosis can be made by a medical provider who is well educated about lymphedema.

33. How can I find a doctor who knows about lymphedema?

If you fail to find a physician in the National Lymphedema Network Directory, you may want to consider checking with a nearby medical center. Some of the larger medical centers have a lymphedema clinical program. Additionally, many cancer centers have experience and expertise with lymphedema that is not widely advertised to the public but is available to patients treated at the cancer center. These centers may be able to direct you to specialized doctors and therapists in your area.

As noted in Question 14, other resources include the schools for lymphedema training. Often, these training programs will offer a listing of specialty providers, both therapists and physicians, who have some expertise in the management of lymphedema.

When you do locate a physician and attempt to make an appointment, it will be important to find out the following information:

- Do they accept your insurance?
- Do you need a referral from your primary physician?

Angiography
(1) A description of blood vessels and lymphatics.
(2) Diagnostic or therapeutic radiography of the heart and blood vessels using a contrast medium to visualize the blood vessels.

- What pertinent medical information will you need to bring with you for the appointment? This may include previous physician consult notes, reports and findings from any scans that have been done, and any blood work that has been done. If you have not had scans or blood work done, do not be deterred from scheduling this appointment; the specialist will recommend these tests if he or she feels that they are necessary.

Do not be discouraged if they are not able to schedule you immediately. Remember that these specialists are quite few in the United States; therefore, their schedules may be very busy. The important thing is that you make contact and establish a relationship with a physician who can oversee the care of your condition.

Jan says:

In my experience, I have found generally that breast surgeons are more aware of lymphedema than general surgeons. Not specialized in cancer surgeries, general surgeons may not have seen as many instances of lymphedema in their patients and may lack training or education in this area.

34. I have never had lymph nodes taken out and have never been treated for cancer, but since a traumatic injury, my legs have been swollen. Can this be lymphedema?

Yes, this can be lymphedema. Traumatic injuries damage lymphatic vessels in many ways. Trauma causes significant inflammation and overloads the lymphatic system temporarily. When the tissue heals, the inflammation and swelling go away and, in most instances, the system returns to normal. However, when an injury is very severe and there is a large amount of tissue damaged, the inflammation may remain for a long period of time. When this is the case, the lymphatic system works at its maximum capacity for as long as it possibly can to alleviate the burden of excess fluid. But, just like any part of the body, the system can only work at its maximum for a certain period of time before it becomes fatigued. When fatigue occurs, the lymphatics become less efficient and are able to remove less fluid. The result is more swelling accumulating in the tissue. As this swelling persists, and the system becomes more fatigued, lymphedema is the result. The back-up of protein-rich fluid eventually causes scarring (fibrosis) in the limbs, and the swelling may be persistent.

Any trauma to a limb that damages the lymphatic vessels will put that limb at risk for lymphedema.

Any trauma to a limb that damages the lymphatic vessels will put that limb at risk for lymphedema. Also, an injury that results in a wound that takes a very long time to heal may damage the lymphatic vessels and cause lymphedema. If the wound is large, deep, and/or circles the limb, there is damage done to the lymphatic vessels, which will impede fluid flow. Even as the injury heals, extensive scarring may prevent fluid from moving and may cause an eventual back-up. The risk of developing lymphedema increases if infection is associated with the injury and if a significant amount of swelling was present at the time of trauma.

If you have experienced a severe injury or extensive surgeries that involved wounds and prolonged healing, and you have swelling that remains in that area, you may want to talk to your healthcare provider about seeing a lymphedema specialist. Persistent swelling after an injury is a sign of lymphatic dysfunction and is treatable with compression and other techniques.

Treatment may help to enhance mobility and joint function and may decrease pain.

35. What if I have had wounds for a long time? Can they cause lymphedema?

Yes, a wound that remains unhealed for a long period of time will eventually cause swelling in the region of the body around the wound. A wound in the tissue creates a constant inflammatory response to help it heal. This inflammation and swelling are due to the lymphatic system being overloaded by the chronic wound, a condition that will eventually deplete the function of the system and may cause lymphedema.

Some wounds, such as diabetic foot or leg ulcers, have a delayed healing time due to circulatory issues. Spinal cord–injured or paralyzed persons can also experience delayed healing of wounds because of poor circulation. Each of these conditions can be associated with the development of edema from various causes. In these instances, the edema initially would not necessarily be lymphedema, but would be related to the venous insufficiency that occurs with poor circulation. However, having venous insufficiency over a long period of time damages the ability of the lymphatic system to work and may lead to lymphedema. This condition is called phlebo-lymphedema, when the veins (phlebo) and the lymphatics are not working.

Excellent nutrition, excellent wound care, and enhancement of circulation are all essential to making sure a wound heals well. Treating any edema, regardless of the cause, will also improve the healing of a wound. Compression bandages or garments are very helpful in alleviating swelling and helping the wound to heal.

Diagnosis and Differential Diagnosis

36. Can lymphedema cause cancer?

In very rare circumstances, a lymphangiosarcoma, also known as **Stewart-Treves syndrome**, may form in association with untreated and long-standing lymphedema. This cancer, once diagnosed, is very aggressive. Typically, it appears toward the far portion of the affected limb as small, purplish papules on the skin that can erode and weep. The exact cause of lymphangiosarcoma in untreated lymphedema is not entirely clear but is likely related to the impaired ability of the limb to filter and dispose of noxious waste materials and viruses within the tissue. The incidence of Stewart-Treves syndrome in the lymphedema population is approximately 2–4%, compared to less than 1% in the general population. It is extremely rare; however, if the limb presents with any of the signs noted here, medical attention should be sought immediately.

37. What is lipedema?

Lipedema is an inherited malformation of fatty tissue. The fat cells in the lower part of the body grow in an abnormal way and are excessively distributed over the lower portion of the body from the iliac crest (near the top of the pelvis) to the ankle bones. The feet are typically spared of the fat distribution. The deposition of the fat is symmetric between both legs. There is a much higher proportion of women compared to men who suffer from lipedema. They will often describe their skin as being very tender and sensitive to pressure, often reporting great tenderness out of proportion to the pressures applied. At times, the upper part of the arms is also involved, but generally the proportions of the person with lymphedema are relatively normal from the waist up.

Lipedema is not treatable with complete decongestive therapy (CDT) techniques (see Question 39). Although the name implies that there is a component of edema in the tissue, this edema is due to the malformed fatty tissue. Therefore, treatment with CDT will not decongest lipedema.

The person with lipedema is vulnerable to repeated trauma to the vessels within the fatty tissue. Without the structural support of **fascia**, muscle, and bone, the superficial lymphatics and blood vessels within the fat are far more susceptible to trauma. Often, these persons bruise easily and experience microtrauma to the lymphatics with minor activity. This makes these persons more vulnerable to developing episodes of swelling. When the episodes of swelling become repeated over time or the swelling persists over a long period of time, swelling will become more static in the tissue. When the build-up of swelling becomes more substantial than what the lymphatic system can manage, a back-up of protein-rich fluid occurs in the tissue. Due to the accumulation of this lymphatic fluid within the fatty tissue, lymphedema may result. This mixed form of swelling includes fluid retention from lymphatic disruption and from persistent inflammation and is called **lipo-lymphedema.**

Lipo-lymphedema presents with chronic, asymmetric swelling in the tissue and is often treated in the same fashion as lymphedema; however, it is more challenging to the therapist due to the intense tenderness and discomfort of persons with lipo-lymphedema. Decongestive therapy will alleviate only the lymphatic overload in the tissue and will not have an impact on the fatty tissue. Therefore, treatment outcomes will not be as substantial when lipedema and lymphedema exist together. Treatment with compression bandaging and compression garments may be difficult for the person

Fascia

A fibrous membrane covering, supporting, and separating muscles.

Lipo-lymphedema

A swelling condition of mixed pathophysiological origin that includes symptoms of lipedema and signs and symptoms of lymphatic overload (lymphedema).

Diagnosis and Differential Diagnosis

with lipo-lymphedema. Often, the compression levels needed to manage the condition cannot be tolerated by the patient; therefore, compression is only minimally effective at managing the swelling. Patients who present with a combination of lipedema and lymphedema should receive decongestive therapy including MLD, compression interventions, exercise, and skin care; however, the expectations of the amount of decongestion that will be achieved should be altered from what is expected when treating lymphedema.

PART FOUR

Treatment of Lymphedema

What is complete decongestive therapy?

How long will I have to go to therapy?

What are compression garments, and when should they be used?

More . . .

38. Is there treatment for lymphedema?

Yes. If lymphedema is present in any region of the body, it can be effectively treated using a variety of techniques. Manual therapy techniques, compression bandages and garments, pneumatic pumps, activity, and exercise are conservative treatments that can be done to help decrease lymphedema. Treatment for lymphedema is best accomplished when these techniques are combined and implemented based on the individual needs of the patient. Successful treatment occurs when therapy interventions are applied correctly by a therapist who specializes in lymphedema management and when the patient is compliant with self-management. Complete decongestive therapy (CDT) is widely accepted as the standard of care for the conservative management of lymphedema and is touted as the most effective conservative therapy intervention (see Question 39). Other treatments that may be used to treat lymphedema include surgery (see Question 42). Surgery may be useful if the condition is not well controlled or if it is very aggressive.

Conservative treatment for lymphedema is the first approach used and is successful in most cases.

Conservative treatment for lymphedema is the first approach used and is successful in most cases. If conservative therapy fails to help a patient, then a different approach may be indicated. However, even when the condition is very advanced, conservative treatment can be quite successful, typically resulting in a 60–70% reduction in the limb volume. Remember, if lymphedema is left untreated, it can get progressively worse over time.

39. What is complete decongestive therapy?

Complete decongestive therapy (CDT), is a specific combination of treatment techniques used in a skilled therapy setting to treat lymphedema (**Figure 6**).

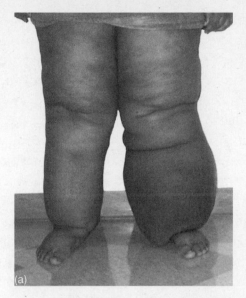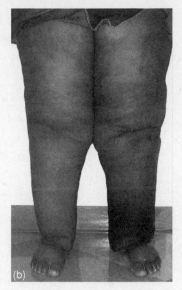

Figure 6   Bilateral lower extremity lymphedema before and after complete decongestive therapy.

CDT includes five components of treatment delivered in two phases. The treatment techniques are very specific in the way they are applied and optimally should be done by a therapist who has received specialty training in decongestive therapy.

In phase 1 of a CDT program, the patient is attending therapy 4–5 times weekly for 60–90 minutes at a time. The treatment includes five main components, designed to be done together. The components of a CDT program are manual lymphatic drainage (MLD), compression bandaging, exercise, skin and nail care. It is also important that, during CDT treatment, the patient learn techniques to care for themselves.

- **Manual lymphatic drainage (MLD)**: MLD is a massage technique that stimulates the lymphatic system by moving fluid away from the swollen areas of the body and toward the healthy regions. When the techniques are applied correctly, the lymphatic system can work more effectively. MLD requires specific hand strokes that are applied to the body in a distinct pattern and direction to move fluid away from the swollen body region. The massage is very slow and light, using just enough pressure to allow the skin to be gently stretched. Too much pressure or too abrupt motion may make the system work less effectively.

The specific sequence is different for every patient and requires a skilled therapist to evaluate the areas of the body that are healthy and to devise an appropriate plan of treatment. Various factors such as scars, the type of surgery that was done, whether radiation was used, and how easy it is to reach some of the healthy lymph nodes all need to be considered when developing a treatment plan.

Our lymphedema traffic jam analogy from Question 8 helps us understand how MLD needs to be applied. Treating lymphedema in a body region is very similar to how a traffic jam resolves after an accident on the highway. After an accident, traffic may back up on the highway for miles. In order for the traffic to begin moving, the cars at the front of the line must move first so those behind will eventually get to move. There are alternative ramps and highways that the traffic can then take to bypass the region of the accident. We cannot resolve the traffic by pushing the cars at the very end of the line of traffic first. Lymphedema is very similar. We cannot resolve the swelling by just pushing the fluid out of the swollen body region first. We must use MLD to clear and open alternate highways for our fluid congestion to flow to. The healthy regions of the body must be treated first so the traffic has a clear pathway to bypass the congestion.

- **Compression bandaging**: Compression bandages are applied to the swollen limb after the MLD sequence is completed and the system has been stimulated to move fluid. The goal of the bandages is to decongest the limb by applying pressure to the tissue and pushing the fluid through the system. It is important that MLD is done first to prepare the vessels to take up the additional fluid that the bandages will move into the system.

  Compression bandages used in treating lymphedema are short-stretch, non-elastic bandages. The non-elastic nature of the bandage gives it a stronger structure against the limb but also makes it more comfortable for patients to wear for an extended time. Traditional Ace bandages are NOT used in treating lymphedema. They can be harmful if applied to the limb.

  Bandages are applied to create a gradient of pressure so there is more pressure at the far end of the limb and gradually lessening pressure at the upper end of the limb (see Question 50). This gradient encourages fluid to move in the correct direction out of the congested region and into the central regions of the body, which have been prepared by MLD to receive the fluid. Specialty compression foam pieces may also be used in conjunction with the bandages to ensure comfort and adequate distribution of the pressure. Your therapist can advise you as to what type of foam may be best to use with your specific condition.

- **Exercise**: Exercises given as part of the CDT program are for gentle, active motion of the body regions affected by swelling. The movement of the limbs, while bandaged, increases the uptake and removal of fluid from the swollen area. Exercise also helps to encourage fluid movement through the

Treatment of Lymphedema

system. The exercises should be recommended by the therapist as part of the CDT program.

- **Skin and nail care**: Since there is a high risk for infection when a patient has lymphedema, there is a need to take good care of the skin and nails to prevent infection. Moisturizing the skin to prevent dry areas from cracking and breaking open is beneficial. Also, taking care to thoroughly clean any small cuts, burns, or bug bites will help to prevent the swelling from worsening. During CDT, your therapist will do a great deal to teach you about keeping the skin clean, moisturized, and intact to prevent skin breakdown and infection, and further swelling.

During the treatment phase of CDT, the limb will decongest and get progressively smaller. Eventually, the therapist will measure for a compression garment that is appropriately fitted for you and will discharge you from therapy once maximal gains have been made. At this time, you will begin phase 2 of a CDT program, which involves self-care to maintain the gains achieved in therapy. During this phase, you will not be seeing your therapist regularly; rather you will be independently managing your condition. The most effective way to maintain your limb volume after therapy will be to wear a compression garment during the day and to continue with compression bandaging (or an alternative compression device) to sleep in at night. This is the best way to keep the limb under control and prevent a reaccumulation of the swelling.

It is of the utmost importance that you have well-fitting garments and have been taught how to bandage during phase 1 of the program. You will continue to manage the condition independently until you are ready to be fitted for another garment (usually in 6 to

9 months), at which time you will see your therapist and can review how the program is working for you and make any needed adjustments.

Jan says:

CDT was highly effective in reducing the volume of my affected arm. When I had stubborn fibrosis in my elbow area, the therapist used foam and special massage techniques to reduce the accumulation of fluid. During the last part of the treatment phase, my therapist took care of ordering appropriately sized sleeves, taught me how to do self-MLD, and gave me literature on exercises to perform. I borrowed a video from the therapist so that my husband would understand how to massage my back and how gentle he needed to be. When I returned several years later to a lymphedema therapist due to hand swelling, I learned some new techniques and modifications to MLD (such as abdominal breathing and massage) that I could incorporate into my routine.

40. When does complete decongestive therapy not work?

In rare cases, conservative treatment like CDT may not be adequate to decongest and maintain the limb volume. If treatment for lymphedema has been unsuccessful, it is important to evaluate the reason for this. The most common reasons that CDT fails are misdiagnosis of the patient's condition, patient noncompliance with the recommended treatment regimen, and incorrect or insufficient treatment of the patient's condition. When it is determined that treatment is not progressing according to the therapist's plan of care, every effort should be made to evaluate these conditions to determine if changes need to be made in the treatment approach.

If the diagnosis of lymphedema is made incorrectly and treatment for lymphedema is being applied, the desired outcome will likely not be achieved. In fact, the outcome may be harmful to the patient. There are many conditions that may cause swelling in the body, including kidney failure, heart failure, and liver failure, to name a few. The swelling associated with these conditions is not lymphedema. If we attempt to use lymphedema treatment techniques on this type of swelling, the side effects may be harmful to the patient and will most likely be ineffective at reducing the swelling. Also, if an underlying condition, such as cancer or a blood clot, has been missed in the initial diagnosis and the treatment for lymphedema is initiated, the condition is unlikely to respond because the factor causing the swelling has not been identified and eliminated.

Patient noncompliance will also contribute to poor outcomes. If the patient does not keep up with the recommended regimen of maintaining the limb with compression garments and bandages, over time, the limb will respond negatively. Devices such as alternative compression garments (described in Question 58) may be substituted on occasion for the compression bandaging regimen to enhance compliance with the phase 2 program. Patients also need to adhere to a healthy lifestyle to help control their lymphedema. Weight gain is the leading risk factor for the development and progression of lymphedema. If weight is not managed appropriately, the lymphedema will continue to progress and be poorly controlled.

Inadequate treatment for lymphedema will also result in poor outcomes. Patients are encouraged to seek out specialty therapists who have advanced skills in lymphedema management. Therapists are further encouraged to implement a thorough and correct treatment plan. Treatment protocols that are most successful involve treatment sessions occurring four to five times per week over several weeks. If treatment is only occurring two to three times per week, it is likely that the outcomes will not be optimal. In some instances, when lymphedema is very advanced, such a treatment schedule may result in no change in the limb volume. Further, in very advanced conditions, additional aggressive treatment interventions should be employed including the use of additional bandages and specialty foam pieces.

If conservative treatment has failed despite adequate management on the part of the patient and accurate implementation of treatment techniques on the part of the therapist, other modes of intervention may need to be explored.

41. How are pneumatic pumps used to treat lymphedema?

A pneumatic compression pump is an external device applied to the limb that exerts pressure through a pneumatic sleeve (**Figure 7**). The sleeve is filled with air, resulting in pressure against the limb that compresses the tissue and facilitates fluid evacuation.

If pneumatic compression pumps are used, they should be part of a CDT program. In this situation, the pump would be applied after the therapist completes the MLD portion of the session. Following the pump, you would either put on compression bandages to wear until the next therapy session or wear a compression garment.

The pump is less effective if used in the absence of manual lymphatic drainage and compression bandages.

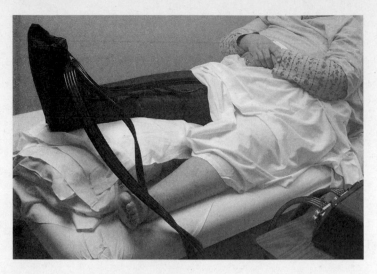

Figure 7   Pneumatic pump therapy.

MLD is needed to open the lymph channels and allow for fluid to flow out of the limbs. Applying the pump without any preparation of the lymphatic system will simply push fluid toward the top of the limb where it will continue to congest. It will not move into the system and be disposed of. Only when the pump is combined with other treatment techniques will the best outcome be achieved.

It is important to do MLD and clear the groin area before using the pump when treating lower extremity lymphedema. If no MLD is performed fluid can built up in the groin and lead into genital causing a disabling condition.

If you are using the pump at home to maintain your limb volume, be sure to do self-MLD first and to put on your compression garment after pump use. When the pump is used alone, it does not maintain the decreased volume over long periods of time. Without compression garments or bandages, the limb will swell back up. Also, if you are using the pump at home, it is important to use the pump according to the pressure, settings, and time that were prescribed for your condition. Often, too much pressure or overuse of the pump can damage the remaining lymphatic vessels in your limb and make lymphedema worse over time. The lymphatic system needs pressure to help it to work, but too much pressure can be damaging.

42. Is there a surgery I can have to treat my lymphedema?

Surgeries to alleviate swelling associated with lymphedema are not common and are only used in very rare circumstances when conservative treatment has not been successful. When a patient is compliant with all phases of complete decongestive therapy yet continues to experience swelling that is not well controlled and/or continues to experience frequent infections, surgery may be an option. However, there are serious side effects to be considered with surgery, and patients must understand that the surgery will not cure them of lymphedema; it will possibly decrease the size of their swollen limb. Additionally, continued lifelong use of compression garments, skin care, and weight management are still necessary after a surgical procedure. While the surgery can diminish the swelling, it does not cure lymphedema.

Surgical procedures are used to reduce the size of the limb by removing the excess bulk of the soft tissue. Lymphedema is a swelling that occurs in the soft tissue, much like a sponge absorbing water. Therefore, in order to remove the swelling, a considerable amount of soft tissue must also be removed. After the limb is surgically debulked of all swollen tissue,

Often, too much pressure or overuse of the pump can damage the remaining lymphatic vessels in your limb and make lymphedema worse over time. The lymphatic system needs pressure to help it to work, but too much pressure can be damaging.

Treatment of Lymphedema

it appears to be slimmer and more symmetrical to the other side.

Many considerations must be weighed before undertaking a surgical procedure. When the soft tissue is removed from the limb, there are numerous lymphatic vessels that are also removed with this tissue. Therefore, the surgical procedure may result in further damage to the lymphatic system. Surgery also introduces the potential for infections and prolonged healing of the surgical incision. Additionally, when surgery is performed, scarring will occur in the tissue. The scar tissue may form a barrier to fluid that tries to move through the remaining healthy lymphatics.

Anastomosis

A natural communication between two vessels; may be direct or by means of connecting channels.

Liposuction

The removal of subcutaneous fat tissue with a blunt-tipped cannula introduced into the fatty area through a small incision. Suction is then applied and fat tissue removed.

The surgical procedures commonly used today include lipo-lymphosuction and microvascular lymphatic **anastomosis**. These procedures require a surgeon to be specially trained in the techniques. Lipo-lymphosuction is somewhat similar to **liposuction** procedures. A cannula (tube) is inserted into the tissue to remove the fatty lymphedematous tissue. The microvascular anastomosis procedures are complicated surgeries that essentially transplant new lymphatics to replace the pathways of the old, damaged vessels. Not every patient will qualify as a good candidate for these procedures. They require that the patient have a specific type of swelling in the limb and that the patient be in relatively good health and be highly compliant with treatment for lymphedema.

Surgical procedures, while successful at debulking the limb, will fail if the patient is not very compliant with ongoing compression interventions after the procedures.

Even after the surgery, the patient will be required to continue wearing compression garments and/or bandages indefinitely to control the limb and ensure that the swelling will not return.

43. Is infrared light effective in treating lymphedema?

Near infrared light therapy (NIR) has been approved for wound care but has not been approved by the U.S. Food and Drug Administration (FDA) for lymphedema treatment. NIR therapy is based on the theory that light-exposed tissue increases available nitric oxide in the area. The nitric oxide theoretically increases tissue repair and may regenerate lymph vessels. The research about NIR in patients with lymphedema does not support that this is a good treatment option at this time, and it is not recommended to be used as a mechanism for treating lymphedema. See **Box 4** for more about novel treatments of lymphedema.

BOX 4	*A Word about "Novel Treatments"*

Be wary of any claims that are not backed by clinical studies. Also, never buy a product without talking to someone on your medical team about the pros and cons and especially the safety concerns with the device. Unfortunately, as in any industry, there are people who are able to make a great deal of money by promising outcomes that they cannot back up. Be an informed consumer to ensure your safety above all else.

44. Is laser therapy effective to treat and manage lymphedema?

The low level laser has been approved in the United States by the FDA for treating lymphedema. The laser uses specific low light beams to change the way our bodies make scar tissue. When lymphedema is chronic, it causes fibrosis (scarring) in the tissue. The laser is shown to decrease the scar tissue in the limb and also decrease the swelling.

Clinical studies from Australia shows that limb volume can be decreased by using the laser device. The response is slow and occurs over a long period of time with repeated use. It is important to note that this device is new, and long-term studies have not been conducted to show its effectiveness in the long-term.

45. Is electrical stimulation useful for treating lymphedema?

Theoretically, some types of electrical stimulation can reduce edema by causing water to be repelled using the magnetic force of the electrical current. This technique does have an effect on edema that is not protein-rich, as the water component of the edema is repelled by the current and encouraged to be removed from the tissue. Lymphedema, however, is a high-protein edema. If the water component of the lymphatic fluid is resorbed, the protein concentration in the tissue increases. The high concentration of protein then attracts more water into the tissue and potentially increases the swelling. Also, the electrical current must be applied for a long period of time for that chemical–ionic reaction to take place and impact the edema. Therefore, electrical stimulation is not a recommended treatment technique for lymphedema.

46. What questions should I ask when I am seeking a therapist?

Treatment and management of lymphedema is best implemented by practicing healthcare providers who have obtained advanced education in specialty techniques. This level of training is sometimes accompanied by a certification. Therapists who choose to become lymphedema specialists should be sought out to provide care for this unique condition. In addition to advanced training, it is ideal that the therapist treating you have experience with patient care directly related to lymphedema and related conditions (see Training Position Paper on NLN Web site).

Sample questions to ask when seeking a therapist:

- Have you received specialty training in lymphedema management?
- How long have you been treating patients with lymphedema?
- Have you worked with patients who have a condition similar to mine?
- Do you use complete decongestive therapy as your treatment intervention?
- Will you do all of my treatment, or are there other therapists on your team?
- Do you have supplies in your clinic, or will I have to order them elsewhere?
- Do you accept my insurance for treatment visits?
- Do you do measurements and fittings for the garments I will need after treatment, or will I need to find another provider for that?
- Do you have a shower facility at your clinic?
- Do you have a support group for patients with lymphedema?

Treatment and management of lymphedema is best implemented by practicing healthcare providers who have obtained advanced education in specialty techniques.

Bonnie says:

The relationship between a patient and a lymphedema therapist is a long-term one. It's important to feel comfortable asking questions, discussing options, and being honest about both compliance and noncompliance. We also need someone who will answer our questions whenever they arise. Fortunately for us, lymphedema therapy is a field that attracts a large proportion of people who are concerned, caring, and generous. I think it helps them when we remember to thank them for the skill and attention they bring to their work—we never know when a word of appreciation might be just what's needed to keep them going in such a tough, hands-on job.

47. What if I can't find someone to treat lymphedema?

We are limited in the number of specialized therapists and clinics in the United States. Often patients have to travel a substantial distance to be treated. Some clinics have a long waiting list, and it may take time to be seen for a consultation and treatment. Contact your closest clinic and find out what the immediate requirements are (e.g., obtaining authorization for consultation and submitting your medical records, including lab work and diagnostic tests), so you can begin the process of gathering all of the necessary information for your consult.

If there is no clinic in your area and traveling is not an option, self-care videos are available and give you an excellent education in the anatomy and basic techniques for self-care. Ideally, you will want to consult with a lymphedema specialist after viewing the video to help you determine which self-care skills are the most important for you to abide by and to help you seek out alternative methods of managing the condition. Sometimes, medical equipment supply companies may be able to connect you with one of the companies that make lymphedema supplies. These companies often have educational materials and information for self-care techniques. Of course, managing your condition should always be done in collaboration with a health-care provider, even your primary care doctor, if no other resources are available. Contact the National Lymphedema Network or go to their Web site (www. lymphnet.org) for information about finding resources.

48. Can a therapist come to my home?

In some instances you may be able to have a therapist come to your home to help manage your lymphedema. Some people are very ill and unable to even walk around their house because their lymphedema is so advanced and their limbs are so large. These people may qualify to receive home-care therapy visits to help them initially manage their lymphedema until it gets to a level where they are more mobile and able to attend regular therapy in an outpatient clinic.

The majority of lymphedema cases will be treated in outpatient clinics. Home-care situations are rare and require that a patient fit a specific set of circumstances. If you have long-term wounds on your legs related to other conditions and also have lymphedema, you may qualify to receive home-care therapy. The last situation is palliative care. When a patient is at the end stages of life, they may be able to receive care in their home from a home-care hospice therapist.

49. What will the evaluation session with the therapist involve?

Your first visit to the therapist will be for an evaluation of your condition. At this visit, you will meet and talk with the therapist about your medical history and the history of your condition. Issues that should be discussed include: how long you have had swelling, how it started, how you have managed it up to this point, including past treatment interventions, and current management strategies. You will also discuss how the condition has impacted your ability to function in your daily activities and work.

The therapist will then perform a physical examination to assess your condition. This will require him or her to test your ability to move your limb(s) and the strength in your limb(s). They will examine the tissue of the body where the swelling exists to note the extent of the edema. In addition, any changes that have taken place in the skin will be closely examined. This examination will require you to disrobe and wear a medical gown so that all areas of the body that could potentially be affected can be examined.

Measurements will be taken of your limb and any associated regions where swelling exists. The measurements are done to determine the volume of your limb. As the limb is treated and becomes smaller with therapy, the volume will decrease. These measurements will help your therapist to determine if the treatment he or she is doing is effective and how much reduction you have achieved with therapy. The measurements may be done by submerging your limb in a tank of water and measuring the amount of water that spills out. Another common way of measuring the limb is to use a tape measure around the limb at set points along its length. Other, more advanced techniques may involve scanning the limb with infrared beams or measuring the limb with an electrical wave.

After this assessment is conducted, the therapist will create a plan upon which you both agree. This plan will include how many days per week and for how many weeks you will be expected to come to therapy. The frequency of therapy depends on how advanced your condition is. The therapist will also recommend specific supplies and materials that you will need to obtain prior to beginning therapy. Once this initial session is completed, you will set up a schedule of therapy visits four to five times per week over the course of several weeks.

50. What will the therapy sessions consist of?

Your therapy sessions will last approximately 60 to 90 minutes. You should wear loose-fitting, comfortable clothing to the first session and should bring all of the supplies that the therapist recommended at your evaluation session. You should expect to be asked to disrobe and wear a hospital or clinic gown. This will give the therapist the best access to all regions of your body. In addition, you will be covered by sheets and towels to maintain your privacy and to keep you warm during the treatment.

The majority of the treatment session will involve manual lymphatic drainage (MLD). MLD is a massage technique specifically designed to stimulate the lymphatic system. Because MLD targets the entire lymphatic system, techniques will be used on your neck, abdomen, armpits, inguinal area, and back, in addition to the limb where you have swelling. Attention to all these areas is necessary to encourage adequate uptake of lymphatic fluid from the swollen body region. See Question 39 for more on MLD.

MLD will be followed by the application of compression bandages to the swollen limb. The bandages have many layers, and several different types of materials may be used.

A layer of lightweight gauze will be used over the limb, followed by many layers of foam padding to protect the skin and allow for an even distribution of pressure. The fingers or toes will be wrapped with a lightweight gauze to ensure that the fluid does not back-up into them. The gauze is very light to allow for easy movement and function. The main component of the bandage structure will be the short-stretch brown bandages. These will be applied in several layers to create greater pressure at the end of the limb and gradually less pressure at the top of the limb. This gradient will encourage fluid to move in the correct direction, up and out of the limb. The bandages come in many different sizes. The smallest bandages will be applied first, and the larger bandages will be applied in sequence as the limb is wrapped up to the top. You will be able to (even encouraged to) move, walk, and do all of your activities while wearing the bandages.

After this portion of the treatment is completed, the therapist will prescribe some exercises that can be done in the therapy clinic or at home. Completing the exercises will help to further enhance the function of the lymphatic system. Once you leave the treatment session, you will be advised to wear the compression bandages throughout the night and into the next day until you return for your next treatment session. The bandages should not be removed until you return for your next session. Your therapist may recommend that you arrive early for your next session so you will have adequate time to unwrap and cleanse the limb before having your next therapy session. This treatment regimen is what should be expected as a standard of care for the majority of patients with lymphedema.

At every therapy session, you may be given handouts and pamphlets describing the treatment and any home activities that you are recommended to complete. You will also eventually begin to learn how to do the compression bandaging for yourself. The therapist will demonstrate the techniques and take you through the process step by step to ensure that you can wrap the limb. Remember that daily attendance at therapy and around-the-clock limb bandaging are temporary treatment interventions that will eventually be altered. Once the limb has been decongested, the regimen will change drastically. So, if you become frustrated with the treatment conditions, remember that eventually you will achieve your goals and will have significantly less constraints on your life.

By the end of your treatment plan, you can expect your limb to have decreased in size by at least 50% in most cases. At this time, the therapist will measure your limb for a compression garment. This may involve many measurements if the garment needs to be custom-sized. If a custom garment is ordered, it may take several weeks for it to arrive. It is important that your therapist measure your limb when it is at its smallest, while allowing enough time for the garment to be ordered, made, and shipped. While you are awaiting the garment, it is vital that you continue daily compression bandaging to keep the limb at a small size until the garment arrives. When the garment arrives, your therapist will ensure that it fits correctly and will review the necessary directions for putting on and taking off the garment, as well as washing and caring for the garment. Your therapist will also review your self-care regimen. The majority of cases will require compression garments to be worn during the day and compression bandages to be worn at night to ensure maintenance of the limb. You should anticipate follow-up with your therapist every 6 to 9 months to reassess the limb and ensure that it is still at an optimal volume before ordering new compression garments.

If you become frustrated with the treatment conditions, remember that eventually you will achieve your goals and will have significantly less constraints on your life.

Bonnie says:

When I started lymphedema therapy it was hard for me to believe it could make any difference. The massage was comfortable and relaxing, but the strokes were kitten-petting gentle—way too soft to do any good, I thought. Wrapping my arm seemed ridiculous, too, with all those layers and layers spiraling up my arm. It certainly stuck out and looked like serious medicine when the therapist was finished, but it also seemed exaggerated—like a cartoon. So I was surprised and gratified that within a couple of days I could see real progress on reducing the swelling and discomfort.

51. How long will I have to go to therapy?

All patients will have a different experience in therapy depending on many factors, such as how severe their condition is, how compliant they are with their care, and how quickly the limb responds to therapy. Mild conditions may only need to have occasional consult sessions with a therapist for education and guidance in self-care and use of a compression garment. Moderate to severe lymphedema will require more extensive treatment. The standard protocol for complete decongestive therapy requires daily treatment until the limb stabilizes. Stabilization may happen over the course of 4 to 6 weeks, or in more severe cases, it may take 2 to 3 months.

The ultimate goal for all patients, regardless of the severity of their condition, is that they eventually become independent in managing their condition. Therapy should be a temporary intervention that optimizes the condition of the limb, alleviates the swelling impairment, and restores function. Regular follow-up visits with a therapist are needed for garment reordering and should occur on average at 6 to 9 month intervals. If problems or complications arise, patients may also need to see the therapist to reassess their condition.

52. What ongoing treatment will I have to be responsible for once treatment is done?

Once the volume of the extremity has decreased to a plateau, the patient is fitted with a compression garment. The goal of the garment is to maintain the extremity and prevent reaccumulation of fluid. Once the garment is received and fitted appropriately, the patient is transitioned into the second phase of CDT— maintenance. Long-term maintenance of the limb can be achieved if the patient is compliant with the use of the compression garment during the day, accompanied by continued bandaging at night (**Figure 8**). At this point, it is important that the patient be independent with self-management, including knowing how to self-bandage, exercise, and use the compression garment correctly.

The long-term outcomes are directly related to the level of the patient's compliance with self-care. Even if your therapist was able to help you achieve a significant reduction in the limb's volume, that volume reduction will be lost if you fail to comply with the self-care program. Additionally, a healthy lifestyle is an important part of a successful treatment regimen. Maintaining optimal body weight is of vital importance to controlling lymphedema.

Even if your therapist was able to help you achieve a significant reduction in the limb's volume, that volume reduction will be lost if you fail to comply with the self-care program.

53. What are compression garments, and when should they be used?

The compression garments are a vital component of managing lymphedema. Compression garments are elastic garments that are fitted and applied to the limb to apply pressure against the tissue. By applying adequate pressure, the garments can help to reduce fluid outflow into the tissue and prevent swelling from occurring.

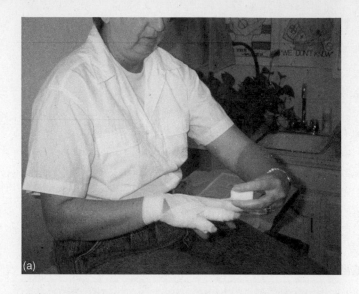

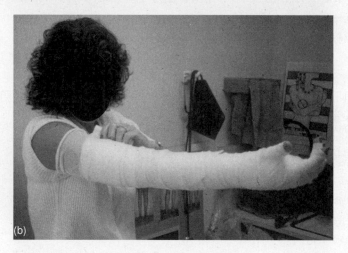

Figure 8 **Self bandaging techniques for the arm.**

Compression garments also enhance the evacuation of fluid by assisting the muscle, and lymphatic vessels, in pumping lymphatic fluid against gravity. In very mild, early cases of lymphedema, the garment may be the primary technique used to treat and maintain the limb volume. In moderate to severe lymphedema, the garments will help to maintain the shape and the size of the limb after optimal decongestion of swelling has occurred.

The upper extremities will require a lower level of pressure than the lower extremities. The lower extremities require greater pressure because of gravity; more pressure is needed to return fluid through the vessels against gravity. Every patient with lymphedema will need to wear a compression garment. The time that the garment is worn will vary depending on the severity of the condition.

54. How difficult are the garments to put on?

In order for the garment to be effective, it must be well-fitted to the limb and translate the prescribed pressure against the tissue. This means the material is fairly tight and will have very little stretch to it, often making a garment challenging to put on and take off. The overall fit of the garment depends on the compression class and style. Higher compression classes are needed for conditions that are more advanced and more aggressive (**Table 2**). When the condition is more advanced, a greater amount of pressure will be needed to maintain the limb. Garments come in various styles (discussed in Question 56), and the choice of style depends on where the swelling is located. Certain styles of garments are easier to put on or take off.

Various tools are available to help with putting on (donning) compression garments. These tools include rubber gloves, silky gloves/socks, silicon gel, or even devices made of parachute material that allows the garment to slide on more easily. These aids are necessary not only to help put the garment on but also to prevent overstretching of the material; they will help

Table 2 Compression Classes and Indications

Compression Class	Level of Pressure	Indications
I	20–30 mmHg	• Mild Upper Extremity Lymphedema • Varicose Veins in Lower Extremities
II	30–40 mmHg	• Most Moderate Upper Extremity Lymphedema • Mild Lower Extremity Lymphedema • Venous Insufficiency
III	40–50 mmHg	• Most Moderate Lower Extremity Lymphedema • Rarely ever used for Upper Extremity Lymphedema
Custom Levels	55+mmHg	• Moderate to Severe Lower Extremity Lymphedema

Source: Standard Classes for Ready Made, Off-the-Shelf Garments.

avoid rips and tears, which may occur if it is a substantial struggle to get the garment on your limb.

There are also different ways the garment can be made to help with donning and placement. Zippers may be put on the garment when it is made for easy donning and removal. Also, when a garment is made in components or separate pieces, it is easier to put on. For example, instead of a full pair of pantyhose, the garment may be made into a pair of thigh-high stockings with an overlying panty-short component to enable easier donning.

The most important point is to be sure that the garment is fitted properly, allowing for even distribution of pressure throughout the limb. Avoid creases in the elbow or behind the knee when putting the garment on.

Important: Create a daily routine to allow yourself plenty of time to put on and take off the garment. Trying different donning aids and strategies will help you find what works best.

55. Should my compression garments be custom-made?

Many different factors need to be considered to determine if your garment needs to be custom-made. These factors include the size and shape of your limb, the needed level of compression, your ability and mobility, and the cost. Each factor should be considered by your therapist in determining what garment choice is best.

If the limb is unusually shaped or excessively long so that a standard-sized garment will not accurately fit, then a custom garment is necessary. Problems may arise if you attempt to fit an unusually shaped limb into a standard-sized garment, as it will be unlikely to maintain the swelling and may do damage to the limb by creating a tourniquet around the misshapen areas.

Patients with more advanced stages of lymphedema will require a higher compression class of a garment. Standard compression garments typically only offer compression up to a moderate level (usually a class III). When a greater class of compression is needed, a custom garment must be made. (See Table 2.)

Custom garments are more expensive than standard garments; therefore cost must be considered when considering a custom garment. The cost of a custom compression garment may be hundreds or even thousands of dollars.

Remember that garments will need to be replaced twice yearly over your lifetime, and an excessively costly custom garment may not be sustainable over that period of time.

56. Are there special garment styles or colors?

Yes, there are various garment styles and colors available. Styles are specific to the body part that needs to be compressed and may be broken into components for ease of fit. Garments for the upper extremity and lower extremity will vary in their styles, and there may be more than one style that is appropriate for each condition.

For patients with arm swelling, the fluid typically extends from the fingers to the top of the arm. In some instances, the shoulder, chest, breast, and back may be involved. Regardless of the location of the swelling, garments are available for almost every part of the body. Styles for the arm include sleeves that extend from the wrist to the armpit and even sleeves with a shoulder cap attached to cover the most upper part of the arm (**Figure 9**). For the hand, there are gloves that cover the hand and fingers or a gauntlet hand piece that covers the palm and back of the hand only. Arm sleeves may be made with a strap that goes around the torso in order to keep it in place or with a silicone band on the top to help hold it up. Compression bras are available to address the swelling that may occur in the breast and chest wall. Often these garments can be customized to account for asymmetry of the breast or chest wall after surgery.

In lower limb lymphedema, patients may experience swelling at varying extents throughout the leg. Many garment styles are available to adequately manage edema throughout the lower limb, including knee-high and thigh-high stockings. These garments can be open or closed

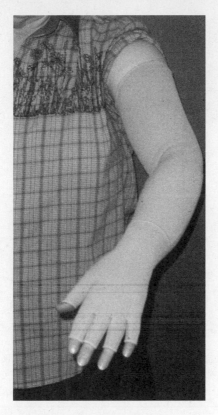

Figure 9   Upper extremity compression garment.

at the toe. If foot and toe swelling exists, a foot cap, which looks like a glove for the toes, should be utilized.

At times, swelling will extend above the groin and into the hip and buttock area, even into the lower abdomen. In this situation a more encompassing garment will be necessary. These garments may include full pantyhose-style or the chaps-style garments, which include a hip component with a belt that attaches around the waist (**Figure 10**). In addition to the many styles that exist, there is a wide range of customization that can be done to the garments. Things such as zippers, straps, waist-bands, and button-fly accessories can be included to ease the burden of wear for the patient.

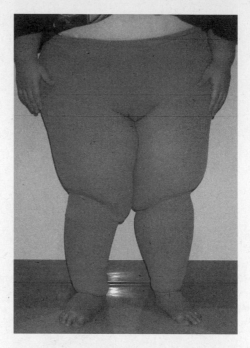

Figure 10   Lower extremity compression garments, custom fit.

In recent years, we have seen a number of companies offer colored sleeves, including various patterns. Many stockings and arm sleeves come in colors, including blue, black, and various skin-toned colors. There is even a company, Biocompression, that offers wildly fun prints and fluorescent colors. The colored garments are typically only offered in the lower levels of compression classes. Some people prefer to wear the colored garments as they can readily match them to business suits, or other work attire. It may help them to feel less isolated.

57. What if I don't bandage every night?

Treatment recommendations should be individualized based on each patient's specific condition. Mild cases of lymphedema may not require compression bandaging on a regular basis or even as a component of care.

For patients with moderate to severe lymphedema, the severity and responsiveness of the swelling will dictate how much compression is needed to maintain the limb. Some patients will require 24-hour compression to ensure that the limb does not refill with fluid. Those patients likely will see an increase of swelling if they do not bandage at night, so it is not a good idea to avoid bandaging.

Another option for nighttime bandaging is the use of alternative garments (see Question 58). These garments are used occasionally instead of bandaging at night. The alternative devices are not intended to replace bandaging but may serve as an adjunct to treatment. Clearly, each patient has different needs. The optimal recommendation is to apply compression bandages to the limb nightly. If you find that you are able to deviate from that protocol without having a negative response in your limb, then you are "learning your limb." Learning your limb enables you to know what your specific needs are and what works best for you.

Jan says:

When I learned about a Reid sleeve (an alternative nighttime garment to bandaging) from an online support group member, I was ecstatic. This compression garment, equipped with Velcro straps, kept swelling down at night without my having to wash bandages every few days, roll them up each night, and use foam. I also experienced less irritation with the Reid sleeve.

58. Are there alternatives to wearing compression bandages and garments?

Bandaging is the gold standard for treating and maintaining lymphedema. However, the task can be difficult for patients to comply with because it is time consuming

The optimal recommendation is to apply compression bandages to the limb nightly. If you find that you are able to deviate from that protocol without having a negative response in your limb, then you are "learning your limb."

and sometimes uncomfortable. It is not realistic for medical providers to believe that their patients will be able to maintain their participation in a daily bandaging routine without fail. Sometimes the bandaging routine may involve both limbs and may include over 20 bandages! There are situations when alternative compression devices may be recommended to help the patient to apply compression to the limb without the time and effort required to bandage. These devices also help to enhance compliance with applying compression to the limb. It is always better to have some level of compression on the limb at night rather than none. If a patient becomes frustrated with bandaging or is simply too tired on some nights to go through the ritual of bandaging, the alternative devices can help save the limb from regressing.

Additionally, there may be other factors that contribute to the difficulties associated with bandaging every night. Elderly and obese patients often have difficulty bandaging their limb. Patients who travel and have a hectic schedule may not have the time to bandage at night; further, they may not be able to pack and carry their bandages on every trip. For young infants in the crawling stage, the bandages come off too easily. Each of these situations is an excellent example of how an alternative compression device can be helpful to apply compression to the limb in the absence of bandages.

There are numerous alternative products on the market (e.g., Reid sleeve, Tribute by Solaris, Jovi, ERX by Telesto Medtech, and Silhouette by CircAid). Some of these products have been on the market for over a decade. They vary slightly but share a common purpose—to provide gentle stimuli to the tissue and to reduce and support the limb. Made from variably shaped dense pieces of foam, they are easy to pull on and off, and they provide great comfort. Some are custom-made while some are bought in ready-to-wear sizes.

In addition to being a supplement to bandaging, these devices can have very substantial uses. Patients sometimes wear them over their garments while flying to provide additional compression. Some patients will use these devices as an extra layer of compression either over or under their bandages. These devices are not intended to fully replace compression bandaging; instead they are best used as an occasional adjunct to the bandages.

Bonnie says:

With two arms and my chest and back involved, there's no way I can wrap every night—and there's no way I want to roll up that many bandages every morning! Instead I wear a special night garment that includes a vest with snap-on sleeves and gloves. They're made of a double layer of soft, stretchy fabric, stuffed with foam chips, and quilted in a pattern that matches the direction of my lymphedema massage. Daytime compression garments depend on the movement of my muscles to help promote lymph flow, but the combination of foam compression and directional stitching keeps my lymphedema under control without depending on my muscle activity to pump fluid; so even when I'm sleeping, my night garments keep the swelling down. In summer I store my night garments in the refrigerator during the day, and the foam holds the cool to help make night compression more comfortable.

59. Can I use a pump in addition to my prescribed treatment?

Some patients use a pump in conjunction with their self-care routine. Continuing to practice manual lymphatic drainage and to wear a compression garment during the day remain vital parts of the self-care routine, and the pump is sometimes added to this routine to enhance maintenance. If a pump fits into your lifestyle and helps you maintain your limb, then using it as a part of the routine makes sense for you. Not every patient will have similar results with the incorporation of the pump, and you should work with your therapist to determine if the pump is right for you.

If you do use the pump, make sure that prior to use, you do your self-manual lymphatic drainage treatment to open the pathways above the lymphedema area and move the stagnant fluid (see Question 41). Doing MLD prior to pump use will help to avoid fluid build-up in the proximal part of the limb (the part nearest the body), as it encourages the entire system to work and take away the fluid pushed out of the limb by the pump.

Important: It is very important that you follow the prescribed pump treatment that was recommended by your therapist. Increasing your pump time and/or the pressure of the pump without direction from your therapist may be damaging to the limb. The pump pressure, if set too high or applied too long, can damage the remaining lymphatic vessels in the limb and have a negative effect.

60. Will treatment for lymphedema cause my cancer to return or to worsen?

Even though the treatment for lymphedema will stimulate the lymphatic system to work more efficiently, there is no evidence that this enhanced system function will cause cancer to return or to worsen in the body. When we diagnose cancer, there is an emphasis on finding cancer in the lymph nodes and on whether cancer has started to move through the lymphatic system. Remember that cancer moves through the bloodstream as well.

When we compare the lymphatic system with the blood circulatory system, both systems are capable of carrying cancerous cells and spreading the disease to other body parts. The circulatory system works at a significantly faster rate than the lymphatic system. The lymphatic system moves only a few liters of lymph fluid each day. There is also evidence that cancer cells found in the lymphatic system may be harbored there and stay there for a long period of time without necessarily progressing and moving through the body.

A study comparing patients who had manual lymphatic drainage to those who did not found that the MLD group did not have a higher rate of developing cancer recurrences. Although treating lymphedema using MLD, exercise, and compression bandaging will promote the movement of lymphatic fluid through the vessels, having treatment for lymphedema is unlikely to cause the cancer to progress or to return.

61. What if I have decided to forgo further treatment for my cancer? How will this affect my lymphedema?

When cancer progresses beyond the point that it is treatable, or when a patient decides to forgo further treatment, there will be an impact on the lymphatic system. When cancer is at its end stage and no treatment is rendered, the cancer cells are taking over various organs and tissues in the body, making it difficult for the lymphatic system to function normally. In these situations, limbs are likely to swell where there has been no swelling before. This swelling is not lymphedema but is related to an overload to the lymphatic system. Lymphedema, when present, will tend to worsen when cancer spreads throughout the body because of this overload but also because in some instances the lymphatic system is impeded upon by a cancer tumor blocking fluid flow.

Lymphedema can still be managed with proper therapy, even if no further cancer treatment is administered. The goals of therapy are adjusted to meet the needs of the patient, who is likely in a **palliative** care stage and receiving no further medical treatment for cancer. Patients in a palliative setting may not be able to attend therapy four to five times per week and may have difficulty tolerating the rigors of an intense complete decongestive therapy program. However, this does not mean they should not be treated. Modifications to the CDT program can prove to be extremely beneficial for patients receiving palliative care. Modifying the bandaging strategies so patients can tolerate the level of compression may be necessary. Modifications may also need to be made to the overall MLD program, as the patient may not be able to tolerate being positioned in ways that enable a full MLD sequence to be performed. These modifications can be made by a skilled therapist. When the program is implemented to the patient's level of tolerance, the outcomes can be incredibly successful.

Even during the end stages of life, there are goals that the lymphedema specialist can help patients to realize regarding pain control, mobility, and independence with self-care. Additionally, encouraging a family member to participate in aspects of lymphedema care may serve to strengthen family bonds at the end of life. When

Palliative

(1) Relieving or alleviating certain symptoms without curing. (2) An agent (e.g., therapeutic procedure, medication) that alleviates or eases a painful or uncomfortable condition.

everyone else in medicine is stepping away from the patient and saying there is no more that can be done, the lymphedema specialist still has a substantial role in helping the patient remain independent and dignified at the end of life.

Bonnie says:

All of us who have had cancer live with the worry that it may return. Adding lymphedema to that picture makes for a nightmare scenario. I've shared these concerns with both my oncologist and lymphedema therapist. There's peace of mind in knowing we're all agreed about the importance of gentle and appropriate lymphedema intervention through-out every stage of my life.

62. Will lymphedema ever go away?

No. Once the lymphatic system has been compromised, there is no way to regrow or repair the system, and if clinically apparent lymphedema occurs, the overload of fluid in the tissue will always exist to some extent. The protein-rich lymphatic fluid will accumulate in the soft tissue much like a sponge soaks up water. Because this fluid is engorged in the tissue, it becomes nearly impossible for the body to ever completely remove all of the excess protein and fluid. If there is an increased level of protein, there will always be an increased level of water being pulled into the tissue by the protein.

Even when the limb is treated and the swelling diminishes to a large degree, there will always be some level of edema that remains in the tissue. The limb will never go back to being completely "normal" and will never look the same as the opposite limb again. This serves as an important reminder that daily self-care is vital to maintain the limb(s). Keeping the limb well-controlled

Once the lymphatic system has been compromised, there is no way to regrow or repair the system, and if clinically apparent lymphedema occurs, the overload of fluid in the tissue will always exist to some extent.

will help to prevent infection, improve mobility, and make the overall maintenance of the condition manageable. You will appreciate your own efforts.

There is evidence that if lymphedema is caught at its earliest presentation, sometimes before there is even visible swelling, it can be alleviated using a lightweight compression garment. This "subclinical" level of lymphedema is defined by sensory changes that patients report feeling, such as heaviness, aching, and tingling. At this level, the body is beginning to accumulate fluid in the tissue; however, it is not at the point where we can visibly see the swelling yet. If treatment is introduced at this level, it may prevent the swelling from progressing to a more advanced, visible stage.

Bonnie says:

It was hard to get my head around the idea that this condition is forever. Other kinds of swelling can be "cured" with time and care, so it doesn't seem fair that lymphedema should be any different. Even after dealing with it for several years, there are days when I can hardly believe it's not going to go away. I've coped with this in a lot of different ways, from ignoring it and trying not to think about it, to crying or raging. Nothing changes the reality, but learning all I can about it so I can keep it in good control has allowed me to take back control of my life. In the process, I've been excited to discover all the new research being done to find better ways to manage lymphedema and, some day, maybe even to cure it.

63. What if I notice a sudden increase in the size of my limb?

Any time a significant increase of your lymphedema occurs very quickly, you should seek a consult with your medical provider. Typically the onset and progression of lymphedema is slow and occurs over a longer period of time. When a quick increase occurs, it usually means something is blocking the system from moving fluid or blood, or something has drastically changed the way your body is managing fluid. Either of these situations warrant a visit to your medical provider, especially if the increase in swelling is accompanied with pain, redness, or warmth to the limb.

A blockage in the system that causes swelling can be attributed to a few different factors. A tumor that is growing in the lymphatic system or near the lymphatic vessels and is pressing against the vessels can block the flow of lymph fluid and cause a quick back-up. If a blood clot is in the vein and blocking blood flow out of the limb, it can cause a quick back-up of blood and result in swelling. These situations will usually cause a quick progression of the swelling and may be associated with pain and redness in the tissue.

An infection in your limb or even elsewhere in your body has a great effect on how your body manages fluid. If you have an infection, you may see your condition worsen very quickly. Remember that infections can spread quickly in people with lymphedema, so it is vital to see your medical provider.

Remember that infections can spread quickly in people with lymphedema, so it is vital to see your medical provider.

If you are fearful about why your swelling has progressed, remember that this is a normal response; your fears should guide you to seeking out a medical consult to determine the nature of the underlying problem. The sooner the condition is diagnosed, the sooner it can be managed, and the better controlled your lymphedema will be.

PART FIVE

Lifelong Commitment to Managing Lymphedema

How frequently do I need to get new garments?

Will my lymphedema get worse as I grow older?

What should I look for to know if something is wrong with my limb?

More . . .

64. What happens after I finish treatment?

After you have finished your treatment, your therapist will provide you with a treatment plan to ensure that you continue your daily self-care. Because lymphedema is a chronic condition, it will require ongoing daily care for the rest of your life. Most lymphedema clinics educate patients and family members in self-care in order to monitor and maintain the affected limb(s) on a day-to-day basis. You will also need to continue to have regular follow-up visits for your condition. It will be important to see a medical provider to ensure that the condition is maintained. You will also need to have new compression garments ordered on a regular basis, usually every 6 months (see Question 65).

Maintaining a healthy lifestyle—including weight management, healthy eating, exercise, and skin care—is important for keeping lymphedema under control.

In addition, maintaining a healthy lifestyle—including weight management, healthy eating, exercise, and skin care—is important for keeping lymphedema under control.

65. How frequently do I need to get new garments?

The life expectancy of garments varies by patient according to the use and care given to the garments. The compression garments used for daily wear will need to be replaced every 6 to 9 months. It is recommended that your limb be reassessed and remeasured each time you need a new garment. Changes in the limb may occur over the time that you are in the self-care stage. Weight loss or gain will change the size and shape of the limb. In addition, as you wear compression garments, your limb will keep a soft and supple texture. Often, as the limb stabilizes, a different compression class will be recommended. Seeing your medical provider will ensure that you are fitted for the correct size, shape, and compression level.

It is recommended that you have two garments at all times so they can be alternated to allow for washing. This practice will promote better life of the garments and enable more regular compression on the limb. Often, once a garment is washed, it may take up to a day to dry because the garments cannot be placed in a hot laundry dryer. Putting your garment in the dryer will damage the elasticity, and the fibers will deteriorate much more quickly. Allow them to air-dry on a towel, avoiding direct sunlight. Having a second garment to wear as the other dries will prevent your limb from going without compression for a long period of time and will also help to prolong the life of the garment.

Jan says:

I wash my compression sleeve every night before I go to bed. It is as routine as brushing and flossing my teeth. I always keep a spare one (an older sleeve that I no longer wear daily) in my suitcase so that if I travel and forget to bring the sleeve that is drying from the night before, I will have two for my trip.

66. How frequently do I need to see my therapist?

Unless complications or concerns arise earlier, you should see your therapist in a follow-up visit every 6 months. At that time, the therapist will measure the limb(s), review any medical changes, and answer any questions you may have. At that time, you also will be measured for a new garment(s).

67. Will my lymphedema get worse as I grow older?

When we get older, we often develop other medical problems, which could influence the lymphedema. Also, like all body systems, the lymphatic system will age and may need additional support, such as stronger compression garments, with age. This reinforces the recommendation that the team of medical providers should be a part of your regular, ongoing care.

New medical conditions may arise and have an impact on how the lymphatic system functions. Conditions that affect the heart, liver, and kidneys may have an impact on how the body manages fluid. Sometimes these conditions can cause an exacerbation of lymphedema as the burden on the lymphatic system becomes greater. Medications may be prescribed for these conditions that may have many side effects, including swelling. If a new medical condition arises or you are placed on new medications, you should follow up with your lymphedema specialist and explain the change in your medical status. These situations may require that you obtain new compression garments of greater compression strength. They may also require that you wear compression more regularly.

Important: Your therapist needs to be made aware of any new medical conditions that arise. This information will assist the therapist in deciding whether to revise your treatment plan as well as in making other decisions that are important to your health. Most importantly, continue your day-to-day self-care, wear a well-fitted garment, and maintain regular exercise.

Jan says:

As I get older, I don't see a significant worsening of my lymphedema. Monthly I check the skin on my affected arm to see if any moles have changed in size, color, or shape, and for other signs of skin cancer. Catching it early will minimize any surgery to remove skin on that limb. The compression garments do not substitute for wearing sunscreen on the limb, but I find that if I wear long sleeves over the compression sleeve, my affected arm is lighter in color than my other arm, even though I wear sunscreen on the unaffected arm. As to drugs, be sure to tell your therapist all the herbs and supplements you are taking, as they might interact with prescription and over-the-counter drugs you are taking for other conditions.

68. Should I have surgery if the lymphedema keeps coming back?

Before making the decision to have surgery, you should consult with your medical team to determine the reason the lymphedema comes back. Rule out possibilities such as recurrent cancer or possibly a tumor blocking the lymphatic vessels. A low-grade infection may exist that is not symptomatic but is creating a higher level of inflammation in the body and causing the lymphedema to be uncontrolled. Medications that have swelling as a side effect may also have an impact on the lymphedema, making it more difficult to control.

You will need to continue self-care for lymphedema for the rest of your life. This means keeping compression garments on daily and wearing regular compression at night. In addition, weight gain will promote the development of lymphedema. If you have fallen away from the regularity of the self-care regimen, the lymphedema may continue to worsen. You may need to reevaluate your level of compliance with the self-care program and determine if there is more you can do to help with upkeep of the condition.

In the United States, surgery for lymphedema is not commonly performed. However, there are surgeons, worldwide, who have developed surgical techniques that are effective, when a traditional program fails, to decrease and maintain the swelling (see Question 42). These procedures require a specially trained surgeon. If you are seeking a consult for surgery, be sure to meet with prospective surgeons and discuss all of the options available to you. In addition, ask them about their level of training with lymphatic surgeries, and ask to see or talk with patients whom they have successfully treated with surgery. It is important to remember that surgery will NOT cure lymphedema. The surgical techniques will decrease the size of the limb and will still require you to maintain a lifelong self-care routine, including the use of compression garments and a healthy lifestyle.

69. What are the signs and symptoms of infection?

The most common infection associated with lymphedema is cellulitis. Cellulitis is an infection of subcutaneous tissues and is most often recognized by a brilliant red color to the skin that feels warm or hot to the touch. Very often patients will describe a period of 24 to 48 hours where they are experiencing flu-like symptoms with a low-grade elevated temperature, achy muscles, and general malaise. If severe, the infection can cause a very high fever with shaking, chills, and sepsis. Cellulitis is a serious condition and requires immediate attention.

The signs and symptoms of an infection are important to look for, as people with lymphedema are at a higher risk for having infections. If you suspect you have an infection, it is best to contact your doctor immediately. If it is after-hours or over the weekend and your doctor is not available, it is best to proceed to the emergency department for immediate treatment. Signs and symptoms include:

- A blotchy redness on the limb
- Redness that becomes progressively worse over the course of several hours
- Redness on the limb that is hot to the touch and may be painful
- New onset of swelling in the limb associated with redness

These symptoms are an indication that there is an infection in the limb. Additionally, if these symptoms are accompanied by a fever, chills, and/or body aches, it is vital that you seek medical attention. Infections associated with lymphedema can progress very quickly and are dangerous.

If the symptoms are present, most often hospitalization and IV antibiotics are necessary. If there is a milder or early onset of cellulitis, very often it can be managed with oral antibiotics as an outpatient.

Bonnie says:

It's one thing to know the signs and symptoms of infection, but it's another thing to act on them promptly when they appear. Unless you've had a bout or two of cellulitis it's hard to believe how serious this situation can be and how rapidly it can spread. Before I had lymphedema, I wouldn't have thought twice about a paper cut or an insect bite.

Now I have to watch even these minor injuries to be sure they don't lead to infection. Nobody wants to go to the emergency room to report redness, warmth, or an itchy rash following something as simple as a torn hangnail, but when there's lymphedema involved, that's actually the smart thing to do.

70. Should I have antibiotics with me if I get infections? And what antibiotics should I have?

If you experience frequent or recurring infections, it may be helpful for you to have a prescription for antibiotics that you keep with you at all times. This enables you to begin the regimen of medication as soon as the first symptoms of an infection are noted. Also, if you plan to travel for a long period of time and/or are traveling overseas, having a prescription for antibiotics with you may prevent an inconvenient and unsafe situation while you are away from home.

If the infection symptoms are relatively mild, most often the infection will be treated with penicillin or a cephalosporin, such as Keflex or Duricef. For patients who are allergic to penicillin or cephalosporin, one of the second, third, or fourth generation quinolones, such as Levaquin or a Ciprofloxacin can be used instead.

A complicated infection with open wounds can be treated with a fourth generation quinolone, such as Avelox. Other antibiotics that can be used include the mycins, such as erythromycin, or the cyclines, such as doxycycline. If there is a suspicion that the infection is due to methicillin-resistant *S. aureus*, very often the patient will need to be hospitalized and treated with vancomycin intravenously. Occasionally, the infections can be managed with oral sulfa drugs instead or some of the newer oral antibiotics, such as Avelox. If there is an element of fungal infection, either as a cause or subsequent to the infection, then topical management with excellent skin care and appropriate topical antifungal medications such as mycostatin can be utilized in conjunction with other oral fungal agents.

Jan says:

Before I travel outside the United States, I have a pharmacy fill a prescription for an antibiotic and take the bottle with me in case I get an infection in a foreign country. When traveling within the United States, I pack a prescription slip that I can take to any pharmacy if I need to have it filled. Certain supplements such as cranberry capsules may help to counter repeated bouts of cellulitis, but check with your therapist or doctor first before buying any. In addition, you might ask your therapist or doctor if you should take an antibiotic as a prophylactic measure before a dental procedure.

71. What should I look for to know if something is wrong with my limb?

Any change in a lymphedematous limb should be assessed carefully. It is worrisome if a limb suddenly becomes more difficult to manage and becomes progressively larger. There can be many reasons for concern that need to be assessed. If the limb becomes red and hot, if there is an increase in pain, or if the swelling progresses rapidly, the situation should be monitored carefully. If the symptoms persist, seek out a consult with your medical provider. If any blistering or open areas occur on the affected limb, it should be carefully cleaned and dressed and watched for any sign of infection.

Any change in a lymphedematous limb should be assessed carefully. It is worrisome if a limb suddenly becomes more difficult to manage and becomes progressively larger.

72. What should I watch for to know if an infection is worsening?

It is important to have baseline measurements of both limbs to know what your normal limb difference is. Measuring the limb on a regular basis will allow you to track changes in it. When an infection occurs, there will be an increase in swelling and likely redness on the limb. As the infection is treated and begins to go away, the redness will start to go away and the excess swelling will begin to go down. If the infection begins to return, you will notice that the swelling begins to progress again, rather than improve. Also, the area of redness on the limb will get worse rather than better. The limb may also feel firmer to the touch and may be painful.

If you have had a recent infection and have finished your antibiotic treatment, and you still notice that the limb is more swollen, is turning redder, and is painful, you will need to consult your medical provider. Infections in a limb with lymphedema may require stronger antibiotics, and they may have to be taken over a longer period of time than in someone who does not have lymphedema.

73. What if the skin breaks out or a rash forms?

A rash or skin change in a limb with lymphedema may occur for a number of reasons, including excessively dry skin, a sensitivity of the skin to a change in your treatment regimen, or a worsening of lymphedema. A noticeable change in the skin should cause you to consult with your medical provider.

Lymphedema causes changes in the hydration of your skin. The skin may be excessively dry and scaly. If the skin becomes excessively dry, it may be easily irritated or itch. The simple remedy to this situation is to excessively moisturize your skin. Using a moisturizer frequently on the skin will help to prevent excessive dryness. You may need to use a significant amount of lotion on a limb with lymphedema to keep the dry skin at bay. Many moisturizers exist and are effective to manage dry skin. It is advisable to avoid lotions with perfumes or dyes, as they may irritate the skin and negate the moisturizing properties.

Topical irritation of the tissue may also exist with continued bandage and compression garment wear. The compression materials need to be washed after one or two daily uses. They cannot be used indefinitely without cleansing. Doing so may cause significant irritation to the skin. Also, your therapist will advise you in the appropriate padding materials to use under your compression bandages. Applying the bandages directly to the skin, without the proper padding, may irritate the skin. Be mindful of the detergents you use to wash your clothes. Changing your laundry detergent may irritate your skin. Also, changes in your diet may have an impact on your skin. There are some food allergies that will appear as skin irritations. If you are unsure of the cause of your skin irritation, consult your medical provider.

If lymphedema is untreated or undertreated, the swelling will worsen, and the skin can become very thick and scaly. Eventually, it may break, allowing the lymph fluid to leak through the tissue. Advanced lymphedema, also called elephantiasis, is characterized by very thick, scaly skin that often has blister-like areas that may weep fluid. Also, red bumps may arise on the surface of the skin in very advanced cases. These situations will be alleviated when lymphedema is treated.

Jan says:

If my skin in the crease at my elbow is red due to chafing from my compression sleeve, I gently apply Eucerin or CeraVe cream to the irritated skin. It provides great overnight relief. When I developed pressure points on my wrists from my nightly bandages or compression glove, I found that strategically placed foam offered relief from the pain.

74. If I have lymphedema, can I . . .

Shave my legs or armpits?

Maintaining skin integrity and preventing infection are vital to practicing good self-care and essential to helping stabilize the limb volume. Any time the skin is cut or scratched, there is a risk that an infection can occur. Situations will occur when nicks, paper cuts, or even bug bites will jeopardize the integrity of your skin. Whenever the skin is cut or punctured, every effort should be made to ensure that the area does not become infected. This care is also true for shaving the limbs. An area of the limb that may be nicked by shaving presents a place for bacteria to enter the skin.

Whenever the skin is cut or punctured, every effort should be made to ensure that the area does not become infected.

For people who have lymphedema, every effort should be made to avoid producing any open areas on the skin. Lymphedema predisposes an individual to infections because of the protein-rich nature of the fluid accumulated in the tissue. Avoiding shaving may help to reduce nicks and cuts to the skin and may help to reduce the risk of developing an infection. Other means of hair removal exist, including creams and lotions and electric razors, which can be effective without damaging the skin. However these products can irritate the skin and cause inflammation. If you have never used these products before, you should first try them on a region of the body that is not affected by lymphedema to ensure that your skin will not be irritated by the cream or lotion.

In instances of genital lymphedema, it is recommended that patients trim pubic hair and keep this area meticulously clean. Pubic hair may be a harbor for bacteria, as the dark, moist environment is a medium for bacteria growth.

Exercise?

Exercise is recommended for people who have lymphedema. When it is done at the right intensity and frequency and under the right circumstances, exercise can actually help to reduce the volume of the limb. Initially, exercise programs should be supervised by a lymphedema specialist who can guide you in the correct exercises and the safest way to complete the program. Compression should be worn on the limb when exercising. The type of compression will depend on your level of swelling. Most people can exercise with a compression garment. The garment will prevent the limb from swelling during the exercise program. Some people will need to wear compression bandages when exercising. The bandages not only prevent swelling, but, in more severe conditions, they can help to decongest the limb while exercising.

An exercise program should be undertaken with the guidance and supervision of a specialist. It is important to gradually increase the intensity and duration of the exercise program so that the limb does not respond adversely. Every patient with lymphedema has the ability to exercise in a safe manner. Exercises, including jogging, weight lifting, aerobics, tennis, and yoga, are all within the ability of every patient. The most important thing to remember is that every exercise or activity should be started at a low intensity and gradually progress under the supervision of a medical professional. Additionally, steps need to be taken to protect the limb (i.e., wearing compression, keeping the limb clean and free of infection).

Any persistent pain in the limb or any exacerbation of the swelling during or after the exercise program should be closely observed. These symptoms are an indication that the exercise program or activity was too intense. Strategies should be undertaken to reduce the chance of overexerting the limb.

Sit in a hot tub? Get a suntan or go to the beach?

Any prolonged exposure to heat will have an impact on the fluid load that a limb has to manage. A limb with lymphedema has an impaired ability to handle an excess fluid load. Therefore, every effort should be taken to minimize situations where prolonged exposure to heat is experienced. The inflammatory response caused by prolonged heat exposure will increase the fluid load into an already compromised limb and may increase the lymphedema.

If you have the opportunity to enjoy a day at the beach or the pool, don't deprive yourself of the relaxing experience! Just do so in a smart way to protect the limb.

Sun exposure is also dangerous if the exposed skin is burned. This situation not only increases inflammation and fluid load to the tissue during the heat exposure, but the residual burn to the tissue causes an ongoing inflammation and longer term increase in the fluid load.

If you have the opportunity to enjoy a day at the beach or the pool, don't deprive yourself of the relaxing experience! Just do so in a smart way to protect the limb. Wear a high SPF sunscreen to prevent burning of the tissue, and keep the lymphedematous limb out of direct sun exposure. Wearing loose-fitting clothes to keep the limb away from the sun will help to diminish the risk of increasing the swelling.

Get a massage?

Massages are a wonderful way to reduce stress and muscle tension. Many different types of massage exist, and some are very safe to have done when you have lymphedema. Remember that the area of the body where lymphedema exists needs to be protected. If you choose to have a massage, be sure the massage therapist knows of your condition, and ask that the therapist either avoid the lymphedematous area or apply techniques that are very light and supportive of the lymphatic system.

Deep-tissue work and excessive pressure from a massage may harm the delicate lymphatic vessels that remain healthy and viable in the limb. Also, any massage techniques that cause excessive friction on the surface of the skin can cause an increase in blood flow and may increase lymphedema. Scented lotions or oils should also be avoided, as they may unnecessarily irritate the skin.

Ride in an airplane?

Going up in an airplane has an impact on how the lymphatic system manages fluid. When the air pressure is lower around our bodies, there is less of a supportive force against our bodies, which may lead to more fluid escaping into the tissues. It is of great importance that if you have lymphedema, you wear compression on your limb when you fly in a plane.

A compression garment or compression bandages will be helpful to prevent the swelling from occurring during a flight. Also, getting up and moving around during the flight further assists the limb at evacuating the excess fluid from the limb. People with lymphedema should not be restricted from taking airplane flights but should take the appropriate precautions as outlined in Question 17. (See Question 17 for more on flying.)

Have blood pressures taken on my limb?

When the limb has lymphedema, it may be sensitive to significant pressure changes. Having blood pressure taken is a necessary part of a medical visit. When you have lymphedema, you should encourage your medical provider to take your pressure on the unaffected limb. (See Question 18 for more on having your blood pressure taken.)

Have blood draws or get shots in my limb?

If you have lymphedema, it is of vital importance to avoid cuts and punctures to the skin. Maintaining skin integrity will help to prevent infection in the limb. If you have lymphedema, you should not have blood draws or injections done on the limb that is affected with lymphedema. These open areas may potentially encourage an infection in a limb with lymphedema.

Take my medications, like diuretics?

Yes! If your medical condition requires that you take medications, even if their side effects include swelling, you should continue to take them. **Diuretic** medications are needed in many conditions that involve the heart, kidneys, and liver. A diuretic, however, is NOT recommended as a treatment for lymphedema. The protein-rich nature of lymphedema does not respond to the diuretic. If you are taking a medication and the side effects include swelling, you should meet with your lymphedema specialist to determine if you

Diuretic

An agent that increases urine output. Diuretics are used to treat hypertension, congestive heart failure, and edema.

need to alter your self-care regimen to accommodate the additional fluid load. This may mean getting a compression garment that is of a higher compression class or wearing compression bandages more regularly. The additional swelling can be managed by altering your treatment plan.

75. Should I have surgery on my affected limb for another condition?

Although recommendations abound to avoid trauma and injury to your lymphedematous limb, surgery is sometimes needed to alleviate a condition so you can live an independent, functional life. When surgery is to be done on your lymphedematous limb, there are a number of steps you and your medical team should take before, during, and after the procedure that will help to maintain your condition.

Before having surgery:

- You may want to have several therapy sessions to ensure that the limb volume is reduced to its smallest point.
- Be sure to have new compression bandages ready to apply after the surgery.
- Your surgeon may begin a preventive dose of antibiotics.

During the surgery:

- Your surgeon should try to minimize the need for a tourniquet on your limb.
- Once the surgical site is closed, compression bandages should be applied to the limb immediately to prevent the influx of additional fluid.

After the surgery:

- Use compression bandages in the immediate postoperative stages. These bandages are easier to manage than a compression garment. The limb may fluctuate greatly after surgery and a garment that was well-fitted prior to the procedure will not fit well immediately after. Also, depending on the type of surgery, the limb may be quite painful to try to fit into a compression garment.
- Your surgeon may prescribe antibiotic medications for you for a bit of time following the procedure.
- Keep the incision site clean and well protected to prevent infection.
- Follow up with your lymphedema specialist, as you may require additional treatment sessions to help bring the limb back to its optimal condition.

A surgical procedure will result in a slight increase in the lymphedema; however, with the correct oversight and care of the limb, you will be able to regain control over the condition.

Jan says:

Don't let any of this advice discourage you from doing what you really enjoy. When I first was diagnosed with lymphedema, I was overwhelmed by all the things I was told not to do. Over time I learned what would cause my arm to swell and adjusted my lifestyle accordingly. Recently, I climbed a mountain over 10,000 feet, wearing two compression sleeves and a glove, with no lasting swelling. My body can tolerate hot tubs if I keep my affected arm out of the water and don't stay in longer than 10 minutes. I believe moderation and common sense are the keys to anything you do. If you do take any drugs that cause swelling as a side effect, ask your physician if there is a drug alternative that does not cause swelling.

You may be surprised that there are, and at the same time you have educated your physician about lymphedema.

76. Can I go back to work with lymphedema?

Most people who have lymphedema go to work and function normally. The only difference is that you need to follow your risk-reduction practices and pay close attention to your limb for possible changes. There are instances when a person's limb can worsen due to job tasks (such as standing in one place, repetitive motions). If that is the case, you will need a letter from your physician outlining the nature of your condition and requesting that you alter your duties at work to alleviate any activities that may trigger the swelling. It is rare, but there are instances when a patient may go on disability. This usually involves situations in which the lymphedema is out of control, causing recurring infections and significant joint and mobility complications.

Jan says:

After I was diagnosed with lymphedema, I continued to work at an office job. I did not notice any adverse effects from sitting for long periods typing on a computer keyboard. If you have any problems on your job, remember that with lymphedema you may be protected under the Americans with Disabilities Act (ADA). Check with a trusted professional to determine if under that act you are entitled to relief from jobs you can no longer perform.

77. Is there a special diet for people who have lymphedema?

A healthy diet that helps you maintain a normal body weight is ideal. It is also recommended that a diet high in fresh fruits and vegetables be consumed because fruits and vegetables are high in bioflavonoids, which can help reduce fibrosis associated with lymphedema. Bioflavonoids will stimulate **macrophages**, which can reduce the protein content of the lymphatic fluid, thus reducing the pressure that can contribute to fluid accumulation and edema formation in lymphedema. Recommendations include a diet low in salt so that unnecessary additional fluid does not accumulate.

There is some compelling research demonstrating that a diet high in selenium may help prevent progression of lymphedema. There is also some work demonstrating that the American horse chestnut can treat venous disease by mildly sclerosing (hardening) the vein, thus reducing the signs and symptoms of phlebo-lymphedema. Additional research shows that bromelain, which is found in pineapple, can reduce inflammation and swelling associated with lymphedema. It is thought that bromelain works by similar mechanisms seen with the bioflavonoid. The ultimate goal with any diet, however, should be to maintain an ideal body weight. An elevated body mass index (BMI) is very highly associated with more difficulty controlling lymphedema.

Jan says:

I believe those with lymphedema are not on a limited diet. The diet advised for lymphedema patients is one that everyone should adopt. Even for perfectly healthy adults, physicians recommend increasing fiber by eating more fresh fruits and vegetables, drinking adequate water, maintaining an ideal body weight, and reducing salt levels. Adopting such a lifestyle will help not only lymphedema but many other conditions. Since I am a cancer survivor, perhaps I am more acutely aware that what I eat may affect my health. I never rely just on supplements to keep my lymphedema under control. I find that compression,

Macrophage

A cell that has the ability to recognize and ingest all foreign antigens through receptors on the surface of its cell membrane; these antigens are then destroyed by lysosomes.

MLD (manual lymph drainage), and gentle exercises are best in maintaining my ideal arm volume.

78. How will my weight affect my lymphedema?

In the last several years, there has been an increase in the body of literature demonstrating that as weight increases, the incidence of lymphedema increases also. In addition, gaining weight can cause the condition to worsen significantly. There is a very clear association of lymphedema with increased body weight, further, lymphedema will tend to improve with reduced weight and there is new evidence that exercise may benefit lymphedema by increasing lean body mass and decreasing body weight. Maintaining an ideal body weight with good nutrition and exercise is recommended for all patients with lymphedema or at risk for lymphedema.

Maintaining an ideal body weight with good nutrition and exercise is recommended for all patients with lymphedema or at risk for lymphedema.

PART SIX

Psychosocial Issues

Sometimes I hate to bandage or to wear the garment; can I take a break for my mental well-being?

There are times I am so angry and frustrated that I have this condition—is it normal to feel this way?

Are there support groups for people with lymphedema?

More . . .

79. How can I deal with people who constantly ask me about my swollen limb?

Many patients, young and old, are self-conscious about their swollen body region, and often it's not possible to cover it up. If you feel brave, tell the curious person that you had cancer surgery and the swelling developed as a result of lymph node removal. Also let them know that this is a chronic problem you are taking care of on a day-to-day basis and that you are doing very well. Don't be surprised if the person tells you that he or she has a friend or relative who had cancer; you will be able to educate this person about the risk reduction practices to avoid swelling. You may find that your advocacy efforts are well received and that the person asking may have resources to share with you.

If your lymphedema is not from cancer-related surgeries, you can politely answer that your swelling is due to a condition that you were born with and that it is a part of who you are. Teenagers often have difficulty answering these questions in peer groups. Being honest with people may serve to educate friends and peers about the condition. Good friends will tend to rally around you and support you for the person that you are in dealing with this condition.

Bonnie says:

Questions from others about my lymphedema are never routine. I'm never quite ready for them, and I'm tempted to be irritated or offended. Of course I would rather not have a condition that requires so much explanation, but I'm slowly learning to cope with looking different and standing out in public. Adults ask about my lymphedema out of either curiosity or concern, but they really don't want to stand still for a long explanation. In most cases, a brief answer works best, something that reveals only as much as I'm comfortable discussing at the time. My standby answer for curious strangers is, "It's a medical condition." With those who are really interested or concerned for me, I spend more time educating them, and I offer to give them written information or Web sites they can look up if they'd like to read more about it. That way I'm helping promote lymphedema awareness, and hopefully making it just a little easier for others who deal with this.

Children are more fun, with their honest and unexpected questions. Their interest is genuine and they're easy to satisfy with simple, direct answers. I keep in mind that they might be worried it will happen to them, so I reassure them that it won't. Sometimes their parents are embarrassed about their questions and try to shush them, so part of dealing with kids is reassuring their parents that I'm not offended.

80. Sometimes I hate to bandage or to wear the garment; can I take a break for my mental well-being?

Certainly there will be days when you do not want to wear your bandages or sleeve/stocking, especially during the summertime or during certain special events. There are even times when you will likely be frustrated with the process of maintaining compression on your limb. These are all situations in which it is okay to step back from the compression garment or bandages for a short period of time.

For most people, a few hours without compression on the limb will not have a negative effect on the overall volume. If this is your situation, you may be able to leave your garment off if you are attending a dinner party or other event where you don't want to deal with

For most people, a few hours without compression on the limb will not have a negative effect on the overall volume.

the cosmetic effect of your garment. There may even be nights when you can get away with not bandaging and still not see a substantial difference in your limb volume. Every patient responds differently to treatment and to ongoing compression therapy. Some will require very high levels of compression on an almost continuous basis; others will not. Between the absolute and nothing, there is a level that is right for you. You can explore the use of compression on and off your limb to determine what is most effective for your limb and to note how long you can go without compression before you see a change in the limb.

Learning your limb is vital to helping you to best manage this condition over a lifetime. It is nearly impossible to believe that everyone will be 100% compliant all of the time. If you do step away from wearing the compression garments or bandages, understand that there will likely be a response in the limb and that you may have to work more diligently to get the limb back under control. This means you may be able to skip a night of bandaging with no problems, but you may realize that after skipping 2 nights, your garment does not fit as well. In this case, you may have to introduce more continuous bandaging over 1 or 2 days to recover from the small increase in the limb. This is a normal process that you will go through to learn your limb and to help you determine what level of ongoing compression is best for you.

Bonnie says:

Even after several years of coping with compression garments and bandages, I still feel disappointed every time I put them on. Taking a break doesn't always work for me because without compression I swell pretty quickly and then have to scramble to get everything back into control. So I use a variety of coping strategies to get some relief. For instance, I make a special point of enjoying the short periods when I'm out of compression to shower and change clothes. I concentrate on enjoying all the textures I can't feel when I have my gloves on and the temperature of the air around me that I miss when I have to keep my arms compressed all the time. I can stretch that time longer if I keep my arms elevated and don't try to do anything strenuous, so I make it a time to relax and chat, read, or watch TV with my family. Another strategy I use when I'm distressed with the garments is to get busy with something I especially enjoy: working sudoku puzzles or knitting or cooking something special. When all else fails, I simply allow myself some time to grieve, then plan a special treat to reward myself for putting up with it all. My family's patience and respect for my needs really help to keep me on track.

Jan says:

I used to be upset that I could not wear sleeveless dresses to special occasions without being self-conscious about my compression sleeve or swollen arm. Then I learned that I could sport such an outfit for an evening without wearing compression if I compensated for any additional swelling by practicing more MLD (manual lymph drainage) the next few days. Now that I have lived with lymphedema for more than a decade, however, I have decided that long-sleeved tops are just as appealing or fashionable as more revealing clothes, and if I wear my compression sleeve, I will not have to worry about increased swelling. It is a very personal decision but not something to impede one's social life. Also, I remind myself that I am being an adherent patient, as I cannot always comply 100% with the lymphedema "official rules." I can adhere to a program that I can live with and that my therapist agrees will be sufficient, as long as my lymphedema is under control and does not worsen over time.

81. There are times I am so angry and frustrated that I have this condition—is it normal to feel this way?

It is absolutely normal for you to feel this way. It is also not uncommon to feel anxiety and stress over managing the condition, anger over even having lymphedema, or even self-pity. All of these emotional responses are normal when dealing with a chronic condition that will require ongoing, daily care. However, when one emotion, such as anger or self-pity, becomes the central focus of your attention and becomes unmanageable, it is time for you to seek assistance to help cope.

When one emotion, such as anger or self-pity, becomes the central focus of your attention and becomes unmanageable, it is time for you to seek assistance.

Coping strategies can be things you do for yourself individually, things you do with a therapist, or things you can do in a support group. Each of these interventions will have a different impact on how you cope with your condition. Individually, you may try visual imagery or relaxation techniques to alleviate your anxiety about the condition. Therapy sessions with a social worker or psychotherapist may be helpful, as the sessions may give you a different opinion and ideas about how to manage your feelings. Talking about these feelings in support groups, where fellow patients experience the same things you do, is a very helpful way to cope with lymphedema.

Many people have medical problems that need to be addressed on a daily basis, but these problems are not necessarily noticeable. Living with lymphedema is often more difficult because people will notice your condition and may ask you questions. Be strong and take advantage of the situation by explaining what lymphedema is, possibly helping others and even helping yourself (see Question 79).

Bonnie says:

For me, lymphedema has created a whole spectrum of emotions, not only anger and frustration, but also sadness and even shame as well. It's hard to brave public events when I'm already feeling so much conflict inside myself. It's a kind of grief, trying to adjust to the losses that lymphedema brings with it—like the freedom to do as I please without having to think about how it might affect my lymphedema, or to go out in public without looking different. But there are a few positive emotions as well, like pride that I've learned so much about this strange condition and satisfaction that I've managed to keep my lymphedema in good control. I give myself room to deal with the difficult emotions, and I try to notice and appreciate the ones that make me feel good about myself.

Jan says:

It is absolutely normal to be angry at your doctors if they dismissed your concerns or didn't give you the proper advice or risk-reduction practices. I was certainly angry with my surgeon. When I noticed initial swelling in my arm and brought it to his attention 18 months after surgery, he told me that unless my fingers looked like cigars I did not have lymphedema. Even though I lived in a major metropolitan area, I did not find a convenient in-person support group. Online I found a wonderful discussion group of understanding individuals who had the same condition and the same concerns, and offered emotional support as well as practical tips.

82. How can I find clothing that will fit when one limb is so much larger?

One of the biggest challenges facing people with lymphedema, as they try to go about their normal daily lives, is finding clothing that can fit limbs that are two different sizes. This can be both a great frustration and a great financial burden. Not only the size of the limb is to be considered when purchasing clothes, but remember that when bandages are worn on the limb, the size is somewhat greater.

For people with severe arm lymphedema, it often is difficult to wear a jacket or shirt. Some people are fortunate because they can sew and make their own clothing or they find a local seamstress, but the majority of people do not have this ability. The best recommendation is to look for looser clothing and clothes made with a bit of spandex material, as they will have the ability to stretch.

Women who have lower limb lymphedema and need to be well-dressed for their job may opt to wear a long skirt or pants that have an element of stretch to them for easy pull-on over the compression stocking(s). Straight-leg pant styles are best suited to wearing compression garments underneath.

Many patients have unilateral lymphedema, and often the foot/toes are involved, which causes great difficulty fitting into a regular-sized shoe. Fortunately, there are numerous options available. Depending upon the formality needed, companies such as Birkenstock, Clarks, and Croc all make shoes that are adjustable and have a wider bias to them for ease of accommodating a wider foot. Nordstrom will fit feet of different sizes and will allow you to buy a "mismatched" pair of shoes at no additional cost.

83. I don't want to burden my family with having to help me manage this condition. How can I get help?

Because lymphedema is chronic, it will require daily care for the rest of your life. The therapist who treats lymphedema will teach you how to continue your self-care on a daily basis. In the meantime, you might have a spouse or other family member who wants to be part of your daily routine and treatment. This is a wonderful time to share together and enjoy each other's company and, at the same time, be productive in maintaining the limb(s). A good idea is to have a set routine for yourself and have specific things that they are able to help you with. This way there is a feeling of support and no resentment about what they are or are not able to do for you.

Just as there will be times when you will need a break from your condition, so will your spouse or family member. Remember to talk about the situation and the frustrations you are both dealing with. As with any situation in a relationship, there will be ups and downs; the most important thing you can do is communicate with one another. Let them know when you need support and when you can manage alone.

Bonnie says:

I much prefer being the one to offer help, not the one asking for it. So I've had to learn gracious ways to ask for help and—what's even harder—gracious ways to accept it. When asking, it eases the way for everyone if I'm clear about what I need so they don't have to guess. When others have to help me, I make an effort to thank them, instead of fuming about needing them in the first place.

Sometimes my family members and friends need help too— it's hard for them to watch me struggle into compression garments every day or fuss with all the bandages. And it's hard for them to be endlessly patient with the time it takes and the limitations I have. Appreciation and a sense of humor go a long way toward easing some of the difficulties of this awkward situation.

Psychosocial Issues

Just as there will be times when you will need a break from your condition, so will your spouse or family member.

84. When will my limb ever look normal again?

At this point, there is no cure for lymphedema, but fortunately, treatment is available. If the lymphedema is diagnosed in the very early stages, you likely will be able to reduce the affected area to a near-normal size. You will need to continue doing your daily self-care and wearing your compression sleeve. For people with stage 2 or 3 lymphedema, with proper treatment, you will be able to reduce the limb substantially, but not to its normal size. Continue to follow risk-reduction practices and daily self-care. The expectations will be different for every person. Work with your medical team and your therapist to set realistic goals and expectations for how your limb should be maintained when it is at its optimal size.

85. Are there support groups for people with lymphedema?

Support groups play a huge role in the lives of patients with lymphedema, particularly because you often do not receive the education and support from your regular doctors. Since lymphedema continues to be an under-recognized condition and a field that is only known to few, often the support groups can be an excellent source of education too. Support groups exist to cover all causes of lymphedema, so a person with breast cancer-related lymphedema might be sitting next to a mom who has a young infant with lymphedema.

There will always be something to learn from one another and to share. The support groups also help you to keep a balanced, realistic perspective on your condition. Also, there may be support groups for different types of lymphedema. When you contact the leader of the support group, make sure you check to see what the make-up of the group is and if it has a specific purpose. The National Lymphedema Network (NLN) lists groups online (www.lymphnet.org) and in *LymphLink*, their quarterly newsletter. They also have guidelines on how to start a lymphedema support group.

Jan says:

I benefited greatly from an online support group for lymphedema through ACOR (Association of Cancer Online Resources; www.acor.org). Two other great online support groups include www.lymphedemapeople.com and www.lymphland.com. The Lighthouse Lymphedema Network (www. lymphedemalighthouse.org) is a very active in-person support group in the Atlanta, Georgia, area.

PART SEVEN

Genetics and Lymphedema

Is lymphedema a genetic condition?

If I have lymphedema, is it safe to become pregnant?

Are there genetic tests to identify if my child will have lymphedema?

More . . .

86. Is lymphedema a genetic condition?

In the United States, approximately 90% of all lymphedema is acquired, or secondary. The most common causes of lymphedema are surgical or trauma. Worldwide, the most common cause of lymphedema is filarial disease. Approximately 10% of all lymphedema cases in the United States are genetic (**Figure 11**). A variety of genetic abnormalities can result in lymphedema. Some of the most easily recognizable genetic conditions associated with lymphedema are discussed in the following list. (See also Question 4.)

- In Milroy's disease, lymphedema is present at birth, and there is a congenital absence of lymphatic

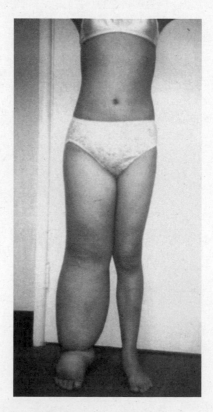

Figure 11   **Primary leg lymphedema in a 7 year old.**

vessels. Recent work on the genetics of this disease indicates that mutations at the VEGFR-3 (vascular endothelial growth factor receptor 3) locus are responsible for the inheritance of Milroy's disease. This is an **autosomal dominant** disease; thus, there is a 50% chance that parents with Milroy's disease will pass the condition on to their child.

- Another widely recognized genetic link to lymphedema is Distichiasis syndrome, in which there are two rows of eyelashes along the posterior border of the lid and associated hyperplasia of lymphatic vessels in the lower extremities, with reflux of lymphatic fluid. This condition can also be associated with problems with drooping eyelids, heart defects, cleft lip and palate, and venous abnormalities. The mutation responsible for this condition has been localized to the FOX C2 gene on chromosome 16.

- There are other identified syndromes such as lymphedema praecox, in which the onset of lymphedema occurs before the age of 35, or, lymphedema tarda, in which the onset of lymphedema occurs after the age of 35. There are often strong family histories of lymphedema in these persons; however, no genetic focus has yet been identified in association with this condition, which on lymphoscintigraphy appears to be due to a lack of distal lymphatics (i.e., lymphatics near the far portions of the body).

- Turner's syndrome is a genetic condition in which females are born with only one X chromosome. Approximately 80% of these infants are born with lymphedema. Interestingly enough, 80% of these children will experience complete resolution of their lymphedema during puberty, which implies a delay in maturation of the lymphatic system as a cause of the lymphedema.

Autosomal dominant

The genetic trait is dominant, meaning a child only needs to inherit the gene from one parent in order to inherit the disease.

- There are other conditions such as Noonan's syndrome, which causes short stature, droopy eyes, low-set ears, and neck webbing, heart abnormalities with lymphedema that is present at birth or shortly after. It appears that lymphedema is related to the presence of a cystic hygroma in utero and is found in instances where the lymphatic vessels fail to mature or are slow to mature. It appears that this condition is related to abnormalities on chromosome 12.
- Yellow nail syndrome is rare and is associated with the presence of yellow nails and upper airway problems, most often with chronic sinus problems, bronchiectasis, and pleural effusions. Lymphedema can be more or less associated with this syndrome. **Lymphography** will typically show mega-lymphatics with pleural effusions (excess fluid around the lungs).

Lymphography

The X-ray examination of lymph nodes and vessels after an injection of contrast medium on the dorsum (top) of the hand or foot.

We are in our infancy in understanding the complexities of lymphatic genetics, and vigorous research is currently underway in this fascinating area of lymphedema research.

87. Is lymphedema in infants treated differently than in adults?

The basic principles of treatment are similar. Every effort is made to maintain excellent skin care, prevent injury to the affected limb, provide movement of stagnant lymphedema, and apply compression as possible. Education is provided for the infant's parents, and they are taught manual lymphatic drainage techniques that can be applied to the child in addition to risk reduction and skin care techniques.

Depending on the location of the lymphedema, compression can be problematic. It is generally agreed that 22- to

24-hour compression is ill-advised in an infant because it can interfere with normal development. It is recommended that when an infant is sleeping, either during naps or at night, a bandage be applied to an affected limb. Garments are not recommended in infants or young children due to the rapidity of growth and the inability to maintain a good fit in a growing limb. Once growth has slowed, sometimes as early as 5 or 6 years of age, garments can be fabricated for the child with the understanding that they may need to be replaced more frequently than in adult patients. Frequent checks with a lymphedema expert throughout infanthood and childhood are recommended so that appropriate compression and devices can be applied. As the child matures, activities such as aquatics and pool therapy can be recommended. In general, contact sports are discouraged for children with lymphedema due to the risk of superficial or deeper injuries and, subsequently, cellulitis.

Bonnie says:

As an adult with lymphedema I can only imagine the challenges that families must face when a child develops lymphedema. It's hard for me to control my frustration when I have to wrap my own limbs, so I can empathize with the stress of wrapping a toddler's restless little legs. My awkwardness in finding clothing styles that work for me and answering the questions that others ask about my condition makes me painfully aware of how hard it must be for young teens with lymphedema to cope with their emerging self-image. But I also know from my own experience that, with the support of their family and the help of a good medical team, these challenges can be met and even turned into strengths.

88. Do I see a pediatrician if I think my baby has lymphedema?

In diagnosing lymphedema in an infant, it would be important to start with the pediatrician and make sure there are no underlying medical conditions that could be resulting in accumulation of edema. Some conditions that can contribute to edema in an infant include kidney disease, heart disease, lung disease, joint dislocation, arthritis, occult fractures, or, very rarely, a deep vein thrombosis or tumor. If the child has been cleared medically and the edema persists, especially if it is unilateral or confined to a portion of the body, the infant should be evaluated by a lymphedema specialist or a vascular anomalies clinic at a children's hospital. A good example would be Boston Children's Hospital associated with Harvard Medical School, and there is also a children's anomalies clinic in Dallas. Please refer to the National Lymphedema Network (NLN) listing of physicians who are experts in lymphedema and would be able to provide diagnostics and assistance in making a definitive diagnosis of lymphedema in an infant (www.lymphnet.org).

In the vast majority of cases, it is safe to get pregnant. With careful attention to compression and a diet with decreased salt, most women do well with pregnancy.

89. If I have lymphedema, is it safe to become pregnant?

In the vast majority of cases, it is safe to get pregnant. With careful attention to compression and a diet with decreased salt, most women do well with pregnancy. This is especially true if the lymphedema is secondary or due to a surgery or trauma and not an underlying genetic cause. In this case, following the usual risk reduction guidelines—in particular, avoiding blood pressure measurements, needlesticks, tourniquets to the affected limb; maintaining good weight; and avoiding salt, extremes of heat, constricting clothing or

jewelry, and trauma to the skin of the affected limb—
are all important in order to avoid associated infection or exacerbation of the lymphedema. (See the
NLN position paper on risk reduction, available at
www.lymphnet.org, for further information on risk
reduction.)

If the lymphedema is due to a genetic cause, it would
be very important for the mother-to-be to have very
close supervision by an informed obstetrician who can
follow the course of the pregnancy and make sure
there are not signs of developmental abnormalities that
can be seen in some of the genetic syndromes associated with lymphedema. For example, webbed necks
associated with Turner's syndrome or Noonan's syndrome are caused by cystic hygroma; this condition can
be seen on ultrasound in utero. If you are uncertain
whether your lymphedema was acquired or genetic, it
would be important to see a specialist in lymphedema
who could help identify the cause of your lymphedema
prior to pregnancy and perhaps have a geneticist
inform you of the risk of passing the condition on to
a child.

90. Are there genetic tests to identify if my child will have lymphedema?

It is not recommended that someone embark on ran-
dom genetic testing if there is no family history or any
presence of lymphedema in the parents; however, if one
of the parents suffers from lymphedema that was not
acquired by surgery, trauma, or some other damaging
event to the lymphatic system and there is a high suspicion for genetic cause of the lymphedema, then consultation with a geneticist is recommended. Depending on
which genetic syndrome is present, the odds of a child

being born with lymphedema can be determined, and decisions regarding whether to get pregnant can be better informed.

91. Our first child was born with lymphedema. Now we are thinking of having a second child. What are the odds that he or she will have the condition?

This is a very complex question and would depend entirely upon what genetic abnormality your child suffers from as a cause of the lymphedema. Some sources of the congenital lymphedema are autosomal dominant, meaning the gene that has led to the first child's condition resides in one of the parents, and there is a 50% chance of it being passed on to the second child as well. Other conditions are linked to the gender of the child; for example, only females will have Turner's syndrome associated with lymphedema. Some conditions have variable expression, and it is not clear what the risk of the condition and lymphedema is. Additionally, there are spontaneous and sporadic mutations that may be responsible for some of the congenital lymphatic syndromes. In the case of one child having lymphedema, it would be advisable to consult a genetic specialist to determine the risk of a second child suffering from lymphedema in the future.

In the case of one child having lymphedema, it would be advisable to consult with a genetic specialist to determine the risk of a second child suffering from lymphedema in the future.

92. Are there support groups for families with primary lymphedema?

While there are many local support groups for lymphedema in general, there are fewer specifically for families with primary lymphedema. The Lymphatic Research Foundation (LRF) is an excellent resource for information regarding support groups for families with primary lymphedema. If no support groups exist, it may be that a chapter could be formed from an existing support group in the area for lymphedema in general. Other resources to find local support groups would include the NLN, Lighthouse Lymphedema Network in Atlanta, Georgia, and treatment centers where therapists who treat lymphedema in your area may be able to help.

93. Where is genetic research done, and how can I participate?

There is a great deal of research actively underway on lymphedema. Much of the research is occurring in laboratories using animal models and looking at cell biology. Several genealogy studies are underway, looking at primary lymphedema. One of the best sources for participating in research regarding primary lymphedema is the Lymphedema Research Foundation. The National Institutes of Health also has listings of research it has funded in the last 5 years regarding lymphedema, and there is active research occurring in Australia, Great Britain, and several sites in the United States. Many of these sources would be able to provide information for ongoing research projects that would be appropriate for you to participate in.

PART EIGHT

Legislative and Reimbursement Issues

How can I get involved with legislation to support lymphedema?

Will my insurance pay for lymphedema treatment?

If my insurance does not pay, is there a way for me to appeal their decision?

More . . .

94. Is there legislation that provides medical provisions for people with lymphedema?

Currently, there is only one piece of legislation that specifically addresses the needs of patients with lymphedema. This is the Women's Health and Cancer Rights Act (WHCRA) of 1998. This act requires that healthcare plans offering treatment for women's cancers also offer coverage for the secondary effects and side effects of the cancer treatment. The act specifically cites that the plan must cover lymphedema.

Further, your state may have laws that direct the insurer to provide payment for treatment that is above and beyond the WHCRA. Check your state's Web site for more information. Also, there may be support groups or advocacy groups in your area that are working toward lymphedema-specific legislation.

95. How can I get involved with legislation to support lymphedema?

Do not be intimidated by the thought that government is big and you are small. Remember that you are important because you vote!

Many organizations have legislative action groups, including the National Lymphedema Network (NLN). There is a need for legislative initiatives at the federal government level, but also at the state government level. Do not be intimidated by the thought that government is big and you are small. Remember that you are important because you vote! Your legislative efforts will be most effective if you are dealing with the officials whom you have a direct impact on electing (or not reelecting).

In your state, you have state representatives and state senators who you elect and who will listen to your concerns. You also have congressmen (or women) and senators whom you send to Washington DC to represent you. These people are the most likely to listen to your concerns about lymphedema-related legislation and to actually respond to your requests as they represent you.

The National Lymphedema Network Web site (www. lymphnet.org) can help you by providing prewritten letters that you can send to your representatives at any level of government. Further, they post action alerts on their Web site when important lymphedema-related issues are being dealt with in government, and they tell you how you can get involved.

96. What is advocacy, and are there advocacy groups for lymphedema?

Advocacy literally means "giving aid to a cause." Advocacy is important to the field of lymphedema because it is a relatively little known condition. In addition, those who do know about lymphedema often do not know enough about the cause, the treatments, and the side effects associated with the disease.

Advocacy comes in many forms. Simply wearing the teal ribbon butterfly pin (the symbol of lymphedema) shows that you are supporting the cause of creating awareness of lymphedema. Advocates can also be educators. Patients who participate in support groups to teach other patients about the risks associated with lymphedema and how to prevent the condition from progressing are advocates. Even simply taking the time to educate the person in line at the grocery store who asks you why you're wearing those bandages on your legs makes you an advocate. Advocacy is about raising awareness and garnering support for this condition.

There are greater roles you can play as an advocate. Taking a position as a community representative on the board of your local hospital will help you to get directly involved in the creation of policies that will have a direct impact on patients and their care. Further, there are many national organizations that foster advocacy for many different conditions. These organizations sometimes have special educational programs to help educate you in the ways of advocacy. Understanding how to talk about the important issues with your legislators and how to interpret current research are topics that organizations may address to help educate you to advocate.

Bonnie says:

Being an advocate is one way of fixing what's wrong about lymphedema. No one warned me about my lymphedema risk or told me how to lower it, so I take every opportunity to educate those with cancer about the simple steps they can take to protect themselves. There needs to be hope of better treatments for this condition, or even a cure, so I've registered at the Lymphedema Research Foundation's patient database, and I keep the promise of research discoveries alive by encouraging research funding through organizations like Avon, Komen, and the Lance Armstrong Foundation. Because it can be difficult to explain my needs to doctors and nurses in an emergency, I've teamed up with others to offer in-service presentations about lymphedema from the patient's point of view for the nursing staff at nearby medical facilities. And since Medicare currently will not pay for necessary lymphedema garments, I've joined in the process of promoting legislation to ensure coverage.

For every aspect of lymphedema that causes us grief, there are ways to bring about the needed changes. Together, we can make the difference in lymphedema.

Jan says:

As a graduate of the NLN Lymph Science Advocacy Program, I can vouch for the fact that a patient-advocate plays a very important and satisfying role. In this capacity, I educate patients, address support groups, educate doctors and nurses in the community, and in general raise awareness of the condition so that others may be helped. I enjoy explaining to curious folk why I am wearing a compression sleeve. In my advocacy role, I have met many cancer survivors who are unaware of the lifelong risk of developing lymphedema and are grateful for information and reminders on risk-reduction practices.

97. Will my insurance pay for lymphedema treatment?

Most insurance providers will provide coverage for lymphedema treatment. The extent of the treatment that will be paid for is variable though. Some will pay for many visits over multiple courses of care, and others will only pay for a select number of visits over a short and defined time period.

Some insurers will require that you have a specific letter of medical necessity from a specialty physician before they will approve payment for therapy. Others will only approve the evaluation therapy session and await the report from the therapist to determine how many visits they will pay for. ALL plans are quite variable, so be sure to check with your specific healthcare plan to determine what you will need before you begin therapy.

Insurance companies are also varied in how much they will pay for supplies and for compression garments. Some companies will cover a set number of garments each year, others will require a letter of medical necessity before they will cover any garments, and still other plans do not cover the cost of supplies or garments at all.

You must be an advocate for your own care. Be certain to get all of the information from your health insurance plan and know exactly what they will pay for and what costs you will have to cover out of pocket.

You must be an advocate for your own care. Be certain to get all of the information from your health insurance plan and know exactly what they will pay for and what costs you will have to cover out of pocket. In addition, there may be co-pays that you will have to cover and/or an overall deductible each year. Having all of the information will help you avoid any pitfalls during or after your treatment. For those who do not have insurance or whose insurance does not cover garments, the NLN offers the Marilyn Westbrook Garment fund; you can download the application from their Web site (www.lymphnet.org).

98. Does Medicare pay for lymphedema treatment or garments?

Currently, Medicare does not pay for compression garments for lymphedema. There is no provision for even a percentage of the cost to be covered by Medicare. There is a current stipulation, as of 2007, if a patient has a chronic wound related to chronic venous insufficiency, then Medicare will only pay for a knee-high garment. A chronic wound is defined as one that has existed for more than 18 months and is a result of the venous stasis condition associated with venous insufficiency.

Many times long-standing venous wounds and edema contribute to the development of lymphedema. Other swelling conditions including lymphedema do not receive any coverage for compression garments or bandages.

Your healthcare payer may require that you have a letter of medical necessity from a specialty provider before they will pay for compression garments (and in some instances treatment). This requirement reinforces the need that you have a medical team made up of lymphedema specialists and conduct regular follow-up visits with them. Working with your medical team enables them to accurately comment on your condition and encourage the provision of medical care and payment for that care.

Bonnie says:

As a lymphedema patient who will one day be on Medicare myself, I worry about how I'll afford my medically necessary compression garments when that day arrives. Working with the National Lymphedema Network's legislative activist, I'm supporting efforts to change that misguided ruling and provide complete lymphedema care for all those who suffer from it.

99. If my insurance does not pay, is there a way for me to appeal their decision?

In most cases, yes, there is an appeal process outlined by your insurance plan. Every company has different stipulations as to how the process works and different paperwork and documents that must be submitted for the appeal process. It is best to talk to your insurance company BEFORE you begin treatment and before you pay out any money for treatment or garments. Knowing up-front, what the insurance company will (or will not) pay for can help you to tailor your appeal.

The insurance company has many different departments, and not all of the departments may have the same set of facts about your condition. When you call to talk to the company, be sure you have all of your medical documents available to reference in your discussion.

Also, make every effort to connect with one person and keep that same person as a contact for every call you make to the company. Often, the first person to answer your call will not be the most helpful to you in navigating the system. The front-line customer service professionals are helpful to answer your basic coverage questions. If your question is more in-depth or if it involves a denial, you will want to seek out someone who is a patient care management specialist or a patient case manager. These individuals are often more knowledgeable in medical conditions and aware of the needs that surround the condition.

Also, your doctor and therapist can play a role in appealing your denial. The doctor may write a letter of medical necessity. This letter outlines your medical condition and why a specific treatment is needed for your condition. With lymphedema, a specialist, such as a physiatrist, vascular specialist, or wound-care specialist may be the best person to help not only oversee the treatment of your condition, but to help with an appeal process. The therapist should be able to clearly document the course of care and the improvements you achieved during therapy. This may include photographs of your limb or body part before and after the treatment, in addition to measurements that were taken throughout the course of your care. These letters from medical professionals help to outline that the course of care was indeed successful and support your appeal process if care is denied.

100. Is there alternative funding for people with lymphedema and limited resources?

Yes, several patient advocacy organizations have special funds that will help to supply financial resources for compression garments and even treatment. These resources are limited and are often provided on an "as needed" basis after a review of your current financial situation. Some organizations such as the National Lymphedema Network, the Circle of Hope, even local branches of the American Cancer Society may have resources available for those who are unable to pay for treatment.

Further, there may be local resources in your community, such as church groups or community outreach organizations (e.g., Kiwanis, Women's Clubs) that may have designated funds to assist people with medical expenses. Also, check with your local hospital, as they may have an auxiliary group that designates funds to assist with resource support.

Alternative funding may be a very helpful alternative for someone on a temporary basis. Remember that lymphedema is a lifelong condition and that treatment and compression garments will be necessary over an entire lifetime. If you are depending on alternative funding, let it be an opportunity for you to begin setting aside your own savings to eventually help take on the cost of managing the condition in the future. Seek out a medical supplier who is flexible and willing to set up a payment plan for you. You may even consider negotiating the rate of your therapy sessions with your therapist if you are paying for treatment out of pocket. Many alternatives exist to help not only defray the costs, but to make them more manageable.

If you are depending on alternative funding, let it be an opportunity for you to begin setting aside your own savings to eventually help take on the cost of managing the condition.

Resource List

General Lymphedema Information

The National Lymphedema Network (NLN)

The NLN is an internationally recognized nonprofit organization founded to provide information for patients with lymphedema.

www.lymphnet.org

The Lymphology Association of North America (LANA)

LANA is a nonprofit corporation composed of healthcare professionals, including physicians, nurses, massage therapists, physical therapists, and occupational therapists experienced in the field of lymphology and lymphedema.

www.clt-lana.org

The International Lymphology Association (ISL)

The goal of ISL is to advance and disseminate knowledge in the field of lymphology and allied topics.

www.u.arizona.edu/~witte/ISL.htm

Lymphedema—National Cancer Institute (NCI)

NCI offers an expert-reviewed information summary about the anatomy, pathophysiology, clinical manifestations, diagnosis, and treatment of cancer-related lymphedema.

www.cancer.gov/cancertopics/pdq/supportivecare/lymphedema/patient

Lymphedema People

Lymphedema People is an information center by and for lymphedema patients that focuses on patients' unique needs, questions, and problems.

www.lymphedemapeople.com

Lymphedema Resources, Inc.

Lymphedema Resources, Inc., is a not-for-profit corporation dedicated to educating, supporting, and assisting lymphedema patients and at-risk cancer survivors.

www.lymphedemaresources.org

Lymph Notes: Lymphedema Information, Books, and Support

This resource offers support for people affected by lymphedema, including patients' families, friends, and therapists.

www.lymphnotes.com

Lymphedema Therapy

Lymphedema Therapy uses the Casley-Smith method of Complete Decongestive Therapy (CDT)/Complex Lymphedema Therapy (CLT) and has helped over 1200 individuals reduce and control their lymphedema.

www.lymphedema-therapy.com

Lymphedema Awareness Foundation (LAF)

This resource offers a continuing educational magazine that focuses on issues and concerns.

www.elymphnotes.org

Lymphedema Therapists, Clinics, Training—LymphSource.com

LymphSource is dedicated to providing education, news, resources, and valuable information for lymphedema patients, therapists, and healthcare professionals.

www.lymphsource.com

Inheritance of Primary Lymphedema

This resource advocates a new understanding of the genetic basis of inherited lymphedema that will provide insights into its treatment and contribute to early identification.

www.pitt.edu/~genetics/lymph/inherit.htm

Lymphedema (PDQ)

This summary provides information about the pathophysiology and treatment of lymphedema.

www.meb.uni-bonn.de/cancer.gov/CDR0000598435.html

The Angiogenesis Foundation

The Angiogenesis Foundation provides patients and their families with up-to-date, expert, and practical information about new angiogenesis medicines.

www.angio.org

Garment and Supply Information

SIGVARIS Corporate

Resource for information on venous disease, compression therapy, and compression stockings.

www.sigvaris.com

Juzo
Manufacturer of gradient compression stockings.
www.juzousa.com

BSN Jobst
Manufacturer of gradient compression stockings, burn scar garments, and adhesive bandages.
www.jobst-usa.com

Smith and Nephew
Resource for research, development, manufacturing, and marketing of devices and products for the fields of orthopedics, wound management, and endoscopy.
http://global.smith-nephew.com/us/

Loehman & Raucher
A leading supplier of dressings, bandaging material, and medical products.
www.lohmann-rauscher.com

Bandages Plus: Lymphedema, Skin Care, Wound Care, and Compression
Supplier of lymphedema and compression therapy products.
www.bandagesplus.com

mylymphedema.com
Supplier of products for treating lymphedema.
www.mylymphedema.com

Lymphedema Products
Supplier of lymphedema treatment supplies, carrying only the most advanced and medically responsible products available for the management of primary and secondary lymphedema, venous edema, and other edemas.
www.lymphedemaproducts.com

Bio-Concepts Custom and Ready-Made Pressure Garments
Manufacturer that has worked closely with lymphedema specialists to develop a protocol for lymphedema garment design that meet the individual's needs.
www.bio-con.com/lymphedema.html

CircAid Medical Products, Inc.
Supplier of products for lymphedema and venous disease compression therapy.
www.circaid.com

Tactile Systems Technology, Inc.
Developer of the Flexitouch system, an innovative, patented medical device for the at-home treatment of lymphedema and chronic wounds.
www.flexitouch.com

JoViPak
Manufacturer of JoViPak compression products for the treatment and management of lymphedema.
www.jovipak.com

Solaris, Inc.
Supplier of custom-made compression garments for lymphedema patients.
www.swellingsolutions.com

Peninsula Medical, Inc.
Manufacturer of fine products for lymphedema and lymphedema-related conditions.
www.noblemed.com

Lymphedema Research Information

The Lymphatic Research Foundation
A nonprofit corporation whose mission is to help identify, support, and promote research into the causes and treatments for lymphedema.
www.lymphaticresearch.org

Lymphatic Research and Biology
A new quarterly peer-reviewed journal, providing an interdisciplinary forum for the world's leading biomedical investigators.
www.liebertpub.com/lrb

National Organization for Rare Diseases (NORD)
Information related to lymphedema, specifically hereditary lymphatic research.
www.rarediseases.org

Lymphedema Family Study
University of Pittsburgh genetic studies project to identify the cause of primary lymphedema.
www.pitt.edu/~genetics/lymph/

Lymphedema Groups Nationwide

Lighthouse Lymphedema Network
Georgia-based education and support network.
www.lymphedemalighthouse.org

Greater Boston Lymphedema Network

Created to supply personal support and share information for
people with lymphedema.

www.gbln.org

Northwest Lymphedema Center

Provides educational material for lymphedema.

www.nwlymphedemacenter.org

West Virginia Lymphedema Network

Members meet as a support group to provide education and guidance on lymphedema issues.

www.wvlymph.org

Lymphovenous Canada

Links people in Canada with lymphatic dysfunction to healthcare
professionals and support groups in their communities.

www.lymphovenous-canada.ca/

Lymphedema Education and Resource Group

Free monthly meetings at the California Pacific Medical Center,
Breast Health Center.

*www.adventurebuddies.net/NEW%20SECOND%20PAGES/
Lymphedema.html*

PLAN: Parents' Lymphedema Action Network

Assists parents of young children affected by lymphedema.

www.lymphnet.org/patients/PLAN.htm

Education in Lymphatic Therapy

The Academy of Lymphatic Studies

www.acols.com

Coast to Coast School of Lymphedema Management

www.lymphedemamanagement.com

HEAT

www.h-e-a-t.com

Klose Training and Consulting

www.klosetraining.com

North American Vodder Association of Lymphatic Therapy (NAVALT)
www.navalt.org

Norton School of Lymphatic Therapy
www.nortonschool.com

The Dr. Vodder School
www.vodderschool.com

Clothing Resources
The Cast Clothing Co.
Custom adaptive clothing manufacturer and retailer for individuals living with a variety of conditions affecting their limbs.
www.castclothingco.com

Catherine's Plus Size Clothing
Offering sizes up to 10X.
www.catherines.com

Just My Size
www.JMS.com

Jesica London Larger Sizes
www.JesicaLondon.com

Aquatic Swimsuits
(800) 235-2156

Markell Shoe Company
Distributing orthopedic footwear, comfort shoes, diabetic shoes, orthotic appliances, surgical shoes, and children's corrective shoes.
www.markellshoe.com
(914) 963-2258

Harry's Shoes (Shoe Warehouse)
Large varieties of adult's shoes and sandals, some in large/wide sizes.
www.harry-shoes.com

Pedifix
Products for problem feet: bunions pads, compression pads, gel toe protectors, and heel pads.
www.pedifix.com

Legislative, Reimbursement, and Healthcare Policy Resources

Centers for Disease Control and Prevention (CDC)
www.cdc.gov

CDC Lymphatic Filariasis
www.cdc.gov/ncidod/dpd/parasites/lymphaticfilariasis/index.htm

World Health Organization
The United Nations public health arm—monitors disease outbreaks and assesses the performance of health systems around the globe.
www.who.int

Global Alliance to Eliminate Lymphatic Filariasis
www.filariasis.org

Centers for Medicare and Medicaid Services
U.S. federal agency that administers Medicare, Medicaid, and the State Children's Health Insurance Program.
www.cms.hhs.gov

Patient Advocacy Foundation
National network for access to care, job retention, appeals, and education for health care. Resources to assist patients in making and defending insurance claims.
www.patientadvocate.org

Patient Services Incorporated
A nonprofit co-pay and premium assistance company for people with chronic diseases.
www.uneedpsi.org

General Cancer Information

National Cancer Institute
Comprehensive cancer information from the U.S. government's principal agency for cancer research.
www.cancer.gov

American Cancer Society
Dedicated to helping persons who face cancer. Supports research, patient services, early detection, treatment, and education.
www.cancer.org

Appendix

157

OncoLink

Comprehensive information on cancer treatments, cancer research advances, continuing medical education, and patient information.

www.oncolink.com

CancerNetwork

Research and opinion by leading oncologists on the screening, early detection, diagnosis, treatment, and prevention of cancers.

www.cancernetwork.com

Meds.com (Cancer Meds)

Offers information and education on prescription medicines (meds) for cancer (including lung cancer, colon cancer, breast cancer, leukemia).

www.meds.com/cancer

National Center for Complementary and Alternative Medicine (NCCAM)

Fact sheet answers some frequently asked questions about complementary and alternative medicine for cancer and suggests sources for more information.

http://nccam.nih.gov/health/camcancer/

Cancer Hope Network

Nonprofit organization that provides one-on-one support to people undergoing treatment for cancer.

www.cancerhopenetwork.org

Center to Advance Palliative Care

Provides healthcare professionals with the tools, training, and technical assistance necessary to start and sustain palliative care practices.

www.capc.org

Children's Cause for Cancer Advocacy

Nonprofit organization that works as a national catalyst to stimulate drug discovery and research for children's cancers.

www.childrenscause.org

Coalition of Cancer Cooperative Groups

Providing the most up-to-date source of cancer clinical trial information for cancer patients, healthcare providers, and advocates.

www.cancertrialshelp.org

National Children's Cancer Society

Dedicated to improving the quality of life for children with cancer by promoting children's health through financial assistance, advocacy, and support services.

www.nationalchildrenscancersociety.org

National Coalition for Cancer Survivorship

A nationwide network of independent organizations and individuals working in the area of cancer support and information.

www.canceradvocacy.org

National Comprehensive Cancer Network (NCCN)

An alliance of 21 of the world's leading cancer centers.

www.nccn.org

General Cancer Research Links

Surveillance Epidemiology and End Results (SEER) Database

Provides cancer statistics.

http://seer.cancer.gov/statistics/

MedlinePlus: Cancer

Source for cancer information through the National Cancer Institute.

www.nlm.nih.gov/medlineplus/cancer.html

National Surgical Adjuvant Breast and Bowel Project (NSABP)

This project has enrolled more than 110,000 women and men in clinical trials in breast and colorectal cancer.

www.nsabp.pitt.edu

ClinicalTrials.gov

Searchable database that provides patients, family members, and the public with information about current ongoing clinical research studies.

www.clinicaltrials.gov

Patient Education Resources for Cancer

Cancer.net—American Society of Clinical Oncology (ASCO) Cancer Foundation

Doctor-approved cancer information from ASCO.

www.asco.org/portal/site/patient

BreastCancer.org—Breast Cancer Treatment Information
Breast cancer information from a nonprofit organization.
www.breastcancer.org

The Cancer Information Network
Articles and resources for cancer patients, their families, and caregivers.
www.thecancer.net

Gilda's Club Worldwide
Resources for women with cancer.
www.gildasclub.org

The LIVESTRONG Global Cancer Initiative—Lance Armstrong Foundation
The Lance Armstrong Foundation unites, inspires, and empowers people affected by cancer.
www.livestrong.org

National Cancer Institute (NCI)
A listing of organizations and groups dedicated to cancer.
www.nci.nih.gov/cancertopics/factsheet/support/organizations

Cancer Resources Specific to Type of Cancer

Malecare
Prostate cancer treatment information.
www.malecare.com

The Oral Cancer Foundation
Oral cancer information and resources for the public, healthcare professionals, and caregivers.
www.oralcancerfoundation.org

Susan G. Komen Breast Cancer Foundation
Dedicated to education and research about causes, treatment, and the search for a cure. Headquartered in Dallas, Texas.
www.komen.org

Ovarian Cancer National Alliance
Mission is to conquer ovarian cancer through uniting individuals and organizations in a national movement.
www.ovariancancer.org

Lung Cancer Online

Cancer and lung cancer organizations. Nonprofit dedicated to basic and clinical cancer research.

www.lungcanceronline.org/sites/cancerorgs.html

Avon Foundation

Committed to the mission of improving the lives of women and their families after breast cancer.

www.avonfoundation.org

Bladder Cancer Advocacy Network

The first national advocacy organization dedicated to improving public awareness of bladder cancer.

www.bcan.org

Inflammatory Breast Cancer Research Foundation

Dedicated to the advancement and research of the condition. Located in Hermosa Beach, California.

www.ibcresearch.org

Cancer Shmancer

Helping to ensure that all women with cancer are diagnosed in stage 1, when it is most curable. Their motto: "Stage 1 is the cure!"

www.cancerschmancer.org

Leukemia & Lymphoma Society

Fighting leukemia, lymphoma, Hodgkin's disease, and myeloma.

www.leukemia-lymphoma.org

Melanoma Research Foundation

Dedicated to finding a cure, this nonprofit also offers information and resources to patients, family, and friends.

www.melanoma.org

Multiple Myeloma Research Foundation

Nonprofit organization aims include fostering a cure by funding research. Addresses the disease, treatment options, and clinical trials.

www.multiplemyeloma.org

National Breast Cancer Coalition

Trains advocates to lobby for legislative and research support for breast cancer.

www.stopbreastcancer.org

National Cervical Cancer Coalition

Information about the organization as well as on the Pap smear, HPV, treatment, and emotional support.

www.nccc-online.org

Foundations to Support Cancer Research

The Breast Cancer Research Foundation

An independent not-for-profit organization whose mission is to achieve prevention and a cure for breast cancer.

www.bcrfcure.org

Gateway Cancer Foundations

Unique among cancer foundations because 99% of every donation goes directly toward research.

www.gatewayforcancerresearch.org/cancer_foundations.cfm

John Wayne Cancer Foundation

Established in 1985, to advance the fight against cancer by supporting research, treatment, and education.

www.jwcf.org

V Foundation for Cancer Research

Charitable organization dedicated to saving lives by helping to find a cure for cancer.

www.jimmyv.org

Prostate Cancer Foundation

Provides prostate cancer information.

www.prostatecancerfoundation.org

The Skin Cancer Foundation

www.skincancer.org

National Breast Cancer Foundation

Official site for breast cancer signs and symptoms, breast cancer awareness, early detection, and breast cancer.

www.nationalbreastcancer.org

Lung Cancer Research Foundation

"Dedicated to discovery" on behalf of lung cancer patients.

www.lungcancerresearchfoundation.org

National Foundation for Cancer Research
Resource for research, related information, news, prevention, and detection.
www.nfcr.org

Bone Cancer Research Foundation
Supports awareness and research into the causes and treatment for bone cancer.
www.bcrfoundation.org

Kaiser Family Foundation
Web site provides in-depth information on key health policy issues including
Medicaid, Medicare, prescription drugs, and more.
www.kff.org

Robert Wood Johnson Foundation
Their mission: to improve the health and health care of all Americans.
www.rwjf.org

Bill & Melinda Gates Foundation
Dedicated to bringing innovations in health and learning to the global
community.
www.gatesfoundation.org

Appendix

Glossary

Anastomosis: A natural communication between two vessels; may be direct or by means of connecting channels.

Angiography: (1) A description of blood vessels and lymphatics. (2) Diagnostic or therapeutic radiography of the heart and blood vessels using a contrast medium to visualize the blood vessels.

Aplasia (referring to lymphatics): The absence of lymphatics. Used to reference a region of the body where lymphatic nodes or vessels failed to develop or grow.

Autosomal dominant (referring to genetic traits): The genetic trait is dominant, meaning a child only needs to inherit the gene from one parent in order to inherit the disease.

Cellulitis: An acute infection of the skin and soft tissue, usually caused by bacteria, characterized by local heat, redness, pain, and swelling, and occasionally by fever, malaise, chills, and headache. The infection is more likely to develop in the presence of damaged skin, poor circulation, or diabetes mellitus. In addition to appropriate antibiotics, treatment includes warm soaks, elevation, and avoidance of pressure to the affected areas.

Chyle: Lymphatic fluid that contains a high level of fat, thereby turning the usually clear lymph fluid white. Chyllous fluid is found in the lymphatic vessels of the abdomen and those that are closely associated with the intestinal tract.

Computed Axial Tomography Scan (CT scan or CAT scan): Computer-generated images of structures within the body created by using multiple X-ray images. The CAT (computerized axial tomography) scan allows us to see soft-tissue and other structures that cannot be seen using X-rays.

Congenital: A condition that is present at birth or very shortly after birth.

Congestive heart failure (CHF): An abnormal condition of impaired cardiac pumping, due to heart muscle tissue that has been injured. Failure of the ventricle to eject blood efficiently results in volume overload, chamber dilatation, and elevated intracardiac pressure. Failure of the left heart causes pulmonary congestion; elevated right heart pressure causes systemic venous congestion and peripheral edema.

Contralateral: Pertaining to the opposite side. The opposite of ipsilateral.

Deep vein thrombosis (DVT): A blood clot in one or more of the deep veins in the legs (most common), arms, pelvis, neck axilla, or chest. The clot may damage the vein or may embolize (or move) to other organs (e.g., the heart or lungs). Such emboli are occasionally fatal.

Diuretic: An agent that increases urine output. Diuretics are used to treat hypertension, congestive heart failure, and edema. Common side effects of these agents are potassium depletion, low blood pressure, dehydration, and hyponatremia.

Doppler ultrasound: A form of ultrasound that can detect blood flow. Commonly used to visualize blood obstructions to blood flow such as blood clots.

Ecchymosis: A bruise that is superficial, caused from bleeding under the skin or a mucous membrane.

Edema: Swelling that is caused by the accumulation of watery fluid in the soft tissues, joint spaces or body cavities.

Elephantiasis: A condition of the skin whereby there is thickening and multiple layers of skin form on top of one another. The skin takes on a scaly appearance and is very rough and thick.

Erysipelas: An infectious skin disease characterized by redness, swelling, vesicles, fever, pain, and lymphadenopathy. It is caused by a species of group A streptococci. Treatment includes antibiotics, analgesics, and packs or dressings applied locally to the lesions.

Fascia: A fibrous membrane covering, supporting, and separating muscles.

Fibrosis: Scarring of the soft tissue of the body. In lymphedema, the scarring is caused by long-standing lymph fluid congested in the tissue. Fibrosis may also be seen in conjunction with radiation therapy when the tissue is damaged and becomes scarred and hardened from the adverse effects of the treatment.

Filaria: A long, thread-shaped worm. In humans, they may infect the lymphatic vessels and lymphatic organs, circulatory system, connective tissues, subcutaneous tissues, and serous cavities. Typically, the female produces larvae called microfilariae. They reach the peripheral blood or lymphatic vessels, where they may be ingested by a blood-sucking arthropod (a mosquito, gnat, or fly). In the intermediate host, they transform into larvae that metamorphose into infective filariform larvae.

Filariasis: A chronic disease caused by the parasitic nematode worm *Wuchereria bancrofti* or *Brugi malayi*.

In the larval stages, the parasite enters the lymphatic system, usually through a mosquito bite, and grows into an adult worm. The worm lives and grows in the lymphatic vessels, making them unable to move fluid and resulting in lymphedema. Filariasis is not typically seen outside of subtropical regions of the world.

Hereditary: Pertaining to a genetic characteristic transmitted from parent to offspring.

Hyperkeratosis: An overgrowth of the horny layer of the epidermis.

Hyperplasia (of lymphatics): Growth of lymphatic vessels that are too large to be functional. The vessels are so large that their ability to move fluid is impaired. The condition is likely to cause lymphatic fluid back-up and lymphedema.

Hypoplasia (of lymphatics): A decrease in the number of lymphatic vessels or nodes that are formed so that they are unable to handle processing a regular volume of lymphatic fluid. The condition is likely to cause lymphatic fluid back-up and lymphedema.

Hypoproteinemia: A decrease in the amount of protein in the blood.

Ipsilateral: Pertaining to the same side. The opposite of contralateral.

Lipectomy: Excision of fatty tissues.

Lipedema: A condition in which fatty deposits accumulate in the lower extremities, from the hips to the ankles, accompanied by symptoms of tenderness in the affected areas.

Lipo-Lymphedema: A swelling condition of mixed pathophysiological origin that includes symptoms of lipedema and signs and symptoms of lymphatic overload (lymphedema).

Liposuction: The removal of subcutaneous fat tissue with a blunt-tipped cannula introduced into the fatty area through a small incision. Suction is then applied and fat tissue removed. Liposuction is a form of plastic surgery intended to remove adipose tissue from localized areas of fat accumulation. There are no health benefits to liposuction, and as with any surgery, there may be risks such as infection, severe postoperative pain, cardiac arrhythmias, shock, and even death.

Lymph: (1) A thin, watery fluid originating in organs and tissues of the body that circulates through the lymphatic vessels and is filtered by the lymph nodes. Lymph enters the bloodstream at the junction of the internal jugular and subclavian veins. (2) The name given to tissue fluid that has entered lymph capillaries and is found in larger lymph vessels. It is alkaline, clear, and colorless, although lymph vessels from the small intestines appear milky from the absorbed fats (chyle). Lymph is mostly water and contains albumin, globulins, salts, urea, neutral fats, and glucose.

Lymph node: One of the many small oval structures that filter lymph and fight infection. Also where lymphocytes, monocytes, and plasma cells are formed. The lymph nodes are different sizes, some as small as pinheads, others as large as lima beans. Each node is enclosed in a capsule. Most lymph nodes are clustered in areas such as the mouth, the neck, the lower arm, the axilla, and the groin.

Lymphadenitis: An inflammation of the lymph nodes.

Lymphangiectasia: Dilatation of the lymphatic vessels (mega-lymphatics).

Lymphangiogenesis: The formation of lymphatic vessels from preexisting lymphatic vessels. When a tumor grows in the body, it signals the lymphatic vessels to grow new vessels.

Lymphangioma: A benign, yellowish-tan tumor on the skin composed of a mass of dilated lymph vessels. The tumor is removed by excision or electro-coagulation for cosmetic reasons.

Lymphangiosarcoma: Malignant neoplasm originating from blood and lymphatic vessels.

Lymphangitis: An inflammation of one or more of the lymphatic vessels, usually resulting from an acute streptococcal infection of one of the extremities. It is characterized by fine red streaks extending from the infected area to the axilla or groin, and by fever, chills, headache, and myalgia. The infection may spread to the bloodstream.

Lymphatic system: A vast, complex network of capillaries, thin vessels, valves, ducts, nodes, and organisms that help protect and maintain the internal fluid environment of the entire body by producing, filtering, and conveying lymph and by producing various blood cells. The lymphatic network also transports fats, proteins, and other substances to the blood system and restores 60% of the fluid that filters out of the capillaries into the interstitial spaces during normal metabolism.

Lymphedema: An abnormal accumulation of tissue fluid in the interstitial spaces. The mechanism for this disease is either impairment of normal uptake of lymph by the lymphatic vessels or excessive production of lymph caused by venous obstruction that increases capillary blood pressure. Stagnant flow of tissue fluid through body structures results in swelling and may make one prone to infection.

Lymphocele: A cyst that contains lymph.

Lymphogram: Also called a lymphangiogram. A radiograph of the lymphatic vessels and nodes.

Lymphography:. The X-ray examination of lymph nodes and vessels after an injection of contrast medium on the dorsum (top) of the hand or foot. Delayed films are taken to visualize the nodes. This technique has been replaced by computed tomography and magnetic resonance imaging.

Lymphorrhea: Flow of lymph from ruptured lymph vessels onto the surface of the skin. Weeping or seeping fluid onto the skin is noted. The fluid is usually clear.

Lymphoscintigraphy: A method used to image the lymphatic vessels and nodes. It involves the injection of a low-level radioactive dye into the tissue at the most distal part of the limb. This allows visualization of the lymphatic system and may highlight areas where the lymphatic vessels are either not working or are absent.

Lymphostasis: Stoppage of the flow of lymph fluid or a build-up of lymph fluid congestion that remains static in one region of the body.

Macrophage: A cell that has the ability to recognize and ingest all foreign antigens through receptors on the surface of its cell membrane; these antigens are then destroyed by lysosomes. Their placement in the peripheral lymphoid tissues enables macrophages to serve as the major scavengers of the blood, clearing it of abnormal or old cells and cellular debris as well as pathogenic organisms. They also release many substances that participate in inflammation, including chemokines and cytokines, lytic enzymes, oxygen radicals, coagulation factors, and growth factors.

Malignant: (1) A condition that tends to be severe and becomes progressively worse. (2) In regard to a tumor, having the ability to invade and destroy nearby tissue and spread (metastasize) to other parts of the body.

Magnetic resonance imaging (MRI): The production of cross sectional images by placing a body part in a static strong magnetic field and analyzing the resonance of hydrogen in various tissues. A computer will generate thin cross-sectional images of the body based on this analysis. This technique is useful for imaging soft tissues.

Melanoma: Any of a group of malignant neoplasms, primarily of the skin, that are composed of melanocytes. They may be sporadic and occur most commonly in fair-skinned people having light-colored eyes. A previous sunburn also increases a person's risk. Any black or brown spot having an irregular border; pigment appearing to radiate beyond that border; a red, black, and blue coloration observable on close examination; or a nodular surface is suggestive of melanoma and is usually excised for biopsy. Melanomas may metastasize and are among the most malignant of all skin cancers.

Palliative: (1) Relieving or alleviating certain symptoms without curing. (2) An agent (e.g., therapeutic procedure, medication) that alleviates or eases a painful or uncomfortable condition.

Papilloma: (1) A benign epithelial tumor. (2) Epithelial tumor of skin or mucous membrane consisting of hypertrophied papillae covered by a layer of epithelium. Included in this group are warts and polyps.

Post-Thrombotic syndrome: A complication that may follow a deep vein thrombosis (DVT) and includes symptoms such as persistent swelling, pain, bruising of the skin, eczema-like skin changes, itchiness, and infections. Also called the post-phlebitic syndrome.

Pulmonary edema: The accumulation of extravascular fluid in lung tissues and alveoli, caused most commonly by congestive heart failure. Serous fluid is pushed back through the pulmonary capillaries into alveoli and quickly enters bronchioles and bronchi. The condition also may occur in barbiturate and opiate poisoning, diffuse infections, hemorrhagic pancreatitis, renal failure, or after a stroke, inhalation of irritating gases, and rapid administration of whole blood, plasma, serum albumin, or intravenous fluids.

Spiral computed tomography (CT) scan: A technique that is performed by moving the patient continuously through the scanner and produces a more rapid and detailed scan of internal structures. This technique is useful for trauma patients and for diagnosing pulmonary emboli.

Stewart-Treves syndrome: Inflammation of a vein in conjunction with the formation of a thrombus. It usually occurs in an extremity, most frequently a leg. The therapeutic goal is to prevent a thrombus from becoming an embolus that may reach the lung. The anticoagulant heparin is used but requires careful monitoring of the patient's response. Therapy may also include ligation of the vein proximal to the thrombus to prevent pulmonary embolism.

Ultrafiltration: Filtration of a colloidal substance in which the dispersed particles, but not the liquid, are held back.

Index

Index

Index